The Treatise on Aromatic Plants

The Treatise on Aromatic Plants

R.C. Upadhyaya

ANMOL PUBLICATIONS PVT. LTD.
NEW DELHI-110 002 (INDIA)

ANMOL PUBLICATIONS PVT. LTD.
H.O.: 4374/4B, Ansari Road, Darya Ganj,
New Delhi-110 002 (India)
Ph.: 23278000, 23261597

B.O.: No. 1015, Ist Main Road, BSK IIIrd Stage
IIIrd Phase, IIIrd Block
Bangalore - 560 085 (India)
Visit us at: www.anmolpublications.com

The Treatise on Aromatic Plants

First Published, 2008

ISBN 978-81-261-3422-9

PRINTED IN INDIA

Printed at Mehra Offset Press, Delhi.

Contents

Preface

Horticulture has a special significance for the economic development. Most of the people, though hard working and face the calamities of nature and live in harsh conditions, yet produce lot of fruits, vegetables and other flowering and ornamental plants including the medicinal and aromatic plants. In order to increase the productivity of horticultural crops growers must take the advantage of the expertise of scientists. Keeping this idea in focus, the present work has been compiled which contains experiences of the experts and related people. The volumes cover advances in strategies, production, plant protection, value addition and other important areas of horticulture development.

The Encyclopaedia provides practical information on production technologies of tropical and subtropical fruits as well as plantation crops and horticultural nursery. Post-harvest management, marketing and export trends have been furnished for guidance. It also presents most realistic cost estimates and returns from cultivation of such crops. The volumes aim at viewing commercial prospects for horticulture. It has been carefully designed to meet the queries of intending investors, financial institutes, creditors, traders and growers engaged in dealing with horticultural crops. Further it will serve the purpose reference books to students, academicians and related people.

R.C. Upadhyaya

Types of Aromatic Plants

Aromatic Fire-cured smoking tobacco is a robust variety of tobacco used as a condimental for pipe blends. It is cured by smoking over gentle fires. In the United States, it is grown in the western part of Tennessee, Western Kentucky and in Virginia. Fire-cured tobacco grown in Kentucky and Tennessee is used in some chewing tobaccos, moist snuff, some cigarettes and as a condiment leaf in pipe tobacco blends. It has a rich, slightly floral taste, and adds body and aroma to the blend.

Another fire-cured tobacco is "Latakia" and is produced from oriental varieties of *N. tabacum*. The leaves are cured and smoked over smoldering fires of local hardwoods and aromatic shrubs in Cyprus and Syria. Latakia has a pronounced flavour and a very distinctive smoky aroma, and is used in Balkan and English-style pipe tobacco blends.

Brightleaf Tobacco

Brightleaf is commonly known as "Virginia tobacco", often regardless of which state they are planted. Prior to the American Civil War, most tobacco grown in the US was fire-cured dark-leaf. This type of tobacco was planted in fertile lowlands, used a robust variety of leaf, and was either fire cured or air cured.

Sometime after the War of 1812, demand for a milder, lighter, more aromatic tobacco arose. Ohio, Pennsylvania and Maryland all innovated quite a bit with milder varieties of the tobacco plant. Farmers around the country experimented with different curing processes. But the breakthrough didn't come until around 1839. Brightleaf tobacco leaf ready for harvest. When it turns yellow-green the sugar content is at its peak, and it will cure to a deep golden colour with mild taste.The leaves are harvested progressively up the stem from the base, as they ripen.

It had been noticed for centuries that sandy, highland soil produced thinner, weaker plants. Captain Abisha Slade, of Caswell County, North Carolina had a good deal of infertile, sandy soil, and planted the new "gold-leaf" varieties on it. Slade owned a slave, Stephen, who around 1839 accidentally produced the first real bright tobacco. He used charcoal to restart a fire used to cure the crop. The surge of heat turned the leaves yellow. Using that discovery, Slade developed a system for producing bright tobacco, cultivating on poorer soils and using charcoal for heat-curing.

Slade made many public appearances to share the bright-leaf process with other farmers. Prosperous and outgoing, he built a brick house in Yanceyville, North Carolina, and at one time had many servants.

News spread through the area pretty quickly. The infertile sandy soil of the Appalachian piedmont was suddenly profitable, and people rapidly developed flue-curing techniques, a more efficient way of smoke-free curing. Farmers discovered that Bright leaf tobacco needs thin, starved soil, and those who could not grow other crops found that they could grow tobacco. Formerly unproductive farms reached 20-35 times their previous worth. By 1855, six Piedmont counties adjoining Virginia ruled the tobacco market.

By the outbreak of the Civil War, the town of Danville, Virginia actually had developed a bright-leaf market for the surrounding area in Caswell County, North Carolina and Pittsylvania County, Virginia.

Danville was also the main railway head for Confederate soldiers going to the front. These brought bright tobacco with them from Danville to the lines, traded it with each other and Union soldiers, and developed quite a taste for it. At the end of the war, the soldiers went home and suddenly there was a national market for the local crop. Caswell and Pittsylvania counties were the only two counties in the South that experienced an *increase* in total wealth after the war.

White Burley

In 1864, George Webb of Brown County, Ohio planted Red Burley seeds he had purchased, and found that a few of the seedlings had a whitish, sickly look. He transplanted them to the fields anyway, where they grew into mature plants but retained their light colour. The cured leaves had an exceedingly fine texture and were exhibited as a curiosity at the market in Cincinnati.

The following year he planted ten acres (40,000 m^2) from seeds from those plants, which brought a premium at auction. The air-cured leaf was found to be mild tasting and more absorbent than any other variety. *White Burley*, as it was later called, became the main component in chewing tobacco, American blend pipe tobacco, and American-style cigarettes. The white part of the name is seldom used today, since red burley, a dark air-cured variety of the mid-1800s, no longer exists.

Shade Tobacco

It is not well known that the northern US states of Connecticut and Massachusetts are also one of the important tobacco-growing regions of the country. Long before Europeans arrived in the area, Native Americans harvested wild tobacco plants that grew along the banks of the Connecticut River. Today, the Connecticut River valley north of Hartford, Connecticut is known as Tobacco Valley, and the fields and drying sheds are visible to travelers on the road to and from Bradley Field, the major Connecticut airport. The tobacco grown here is known as shade tobacco, and is used as outer wrappers for some of the world's finest cigars.

Early Connecticut colonists acquired from the Native Americans the habit of smoking tobacco in pipes and began cultivating the plant commercially, even though the Puritans referred to it as the "evil weed". The plant was outlawed in Connecticut in 1650, but in the 1800s as cigar smoking began to be popular, tobacco farming became a major industry, employing farmers, laborers, local youths, southern African Americans, and migrant workers.

Working conditions varied from pleasant summer work for students, to backbreaking exploitation of migrants. Each tobacco plant yields only 18 leaves useful as cigar wrappers, and each leaf requires a great deal of individual manual attention during harvesting. Although temperatures in the curing sheds sometimes exceeds 100 degrees F., no work is done inside the sheds while the tobacco is being fired.

In 1921, Connecticut tobacco production peaked, at 31,000 acres (125 km^2) under cultivation. The rise of cigarette smoking and the decline of cigar smoking has caused a corresponding decline in the demand for shade tobacco, reaching a minimum in 1992 of 2,000 acres (8 km^2) under cultivation. Since then, however, cigar smoking has become more popular again, and in 1997 tobacco farming had risen to 4,000 acres (16 km^2). However, only 1,050 acres of shade tobacco were harvested in the Connecticut Valley in 2006. Connecticut seed is being grown in Ecuador, where labour is very cheap. The industry has weathered some major catastrophes, including a devastating hailstorm in 1929, and an epidemic of brown spot fungus in 2000, but is now in danger of disappearing altogether, given the value of the land to real estate speculators. The older and much less labour intensive Broadleaf plant, which produces an excellent maduro wrapper as well as binder and filler for cigars, is increasing in acreage in the Connecticut Valley.

Perique

Perhaps the most strongly-flavoured of all tobaccos is the Perique, from Saint James Parish, Louisiana. When the Acadians made their way into this region in 1755, the Choctaw and Chickasaw tribes were cultivating a variety of tobacco with a distinctive flavour. A farmer called Pierre Chenet is credited with first turning this local tobacco into the Perique in 1824 through the technique of pressure-fermentation.

The tobacco plants are manually kept suckerless, and pruned to exactly 12 leaves, through their early growth. In late November, when the leaves are a dark, rich green and the plants are 23-30 inches (600 to 751 mm) tall, the whole plant is harvested in the late evening and hung to dry in a sideless curing barn. Once the leaves have partially dried, but while still supple (usually less than 2 weeks in the barn), any remaining dirt is removed and the leaves are moistened with water and stemmed by hand. The leaves are then rolled into "torquettes" of approximately 1 pound (449 g) and packed into hickory whiskey barrels. The tobacco is then kept under pressure using oak blocks and massive screw jacks, forcing nearly all the air out of the still-moist leaves. Approximately once a month, the pressure is released, and each of the torquettes is "worked" by hand to permit a little air back into the tobacco. After a year of this treatment, the Perique is ready for consumption, although it may be kept fresh under pressure for many years. Extended exposure to air degrades the particular character of the Perique. The finished tobacco is dark brown, nearly black, very moist with a fruity, slightly vinegary aroma.

Considered the truffle of pipe tobaccos, the Perique is used as a component of many blended pipe tobaccos, but is too strong to be smoked pure. At one time, the freshly moist Perique was also chewed, but none is now sold for this purpose. Less than 16 acres (65,000 m^2) of this crop remain in cultivation, most by a single farmer called Percy Martin, in Grande Pointe, Louisiana. For reasons unknown, the particular flavour and character of the Perique can only be acquired on a small triangle of Saint James Parish, less than 4 by 10 miles (5 by 16 km). Although at its peak, Saint James Parish was producing around 20 tons of the Perique a year, output is now merely a few barrelsful.

It is traditionally a pipe tobacco, and is still very popular with pipe-smokers, typically blended with pure Virginia to lend spice, strength, and coolness to the blend. Perique may now also be found in the Perique cigarettes of Santa Fe Natural Tobacco Co., in an approximately 1 part to 5 blend with lighter tobaccos. A similar tobacco, based on pressure-fermented Kentucky tobacco is available by the name Acadian Yellow River Perique.

Oriental Tobacco

Oriental tobacco is a sun-cured, highly aromatic, small-leafed variety that is grown in Turkey, Greece, Bulgaria, and Macedonia. Oriental tobacco is frequently referred to as "Turkish tobacco", as these regions were all historically part of the Ottoman Empire. Many of the early brands of cigarettes were made mostly or entirely of Oriental tobacco; today, its main use is in blends of pipe and especially cigarette tobacco (a typical American cigarette is a blend of bright Virginia, burley and Oriental).

Tobacco Products

Snuff

Snuff is a generic term for fine-ground smokeless tobacco products. Originally the term referred only to dry snuff, a fine tan dust popular mainly in the eighteenth century. This is often called "Scotch Snuff", a folk-etymology derivation of the scorching process used to dry the cured tobacco by the factory. Snuff powder originated in the UK town of Great Harwood and was famously ground in the town's monument prior to local distribution and transport further up north to Scotland.

Snuff has been found to be beneficial in some cases of hay fever due to the fact that the snuff may prevent allergens from getting to the mucus membrane within the nose. Most would say, however, that the detrimental effects of Nicotine outweigh the benefits.

Types of Snuff

European (*dry*) snuff is intended to be *sniffed* up the nose. Snuff is not "snorted" because snuff shouldn't get past the nose, *i.e.*; into sinuses, throat or lungs. European snuff comes in several varieties: Plain, Toast (fine ground - *very* dry), "Medicated" (menthol, camphor, eucalyptus, etc.), Scented, and Schmalzler, a German variety. The major brand names of European snus are: Bernards (Germany), Fribourg & Treyer (UK), Gawith (UK), Gawith Hoggarth (UK), Hedges (UK), Lotzbeck (Germany), McChrystal's (UK), Pöschl (Germany) and Wilsons of Sharrow (UK), TUTUN-CTC (Moldova).

American snuff is much stronger, and is intended to be dipped. It comes in two varieties — "sweet" and "salty". Until the early 20th century, snuff dipping was popular in the United States among rural people, who would often use sweet barkless twigs to apply it to their gums. Popular brands are Tube Rose and Navy.

The second, and more popular in North America, variety of snuff is moist snuff, or dipping tobacco (sometimes known as *smokeless tobacco*). This practice is known as "dipping." In the Southern states, taking a "dip" of moist snuff is called "putting a rub in," the moist snuff in the mouth is known as a "rub." This is occasionally referred to as "snoose" in New England and the Midwest and is derived from the Scandinavian word for snuff, "snuff". Like the word, the origins of moist snuff are Scandinavian, and the oldest American brands indicate that by their names. Snuff is also called a "ding" in New England (*i.e.* "Packing a ding"). American Moist snuff is made from dark fire-cured tobacco that is ground, sweetened, and aged by the factory. Prominent North American brands are Copenhagen, Skoal, Timber Wolf, Chisholm, Grizzly, and Kodiak. American moist snus tends to be dipped.

Some modern *smokeless tobacco* brands, such as Kodiak, have an aggressive nicotine delivery. This is accomplished with a higher dose of nicotine than cigarettes, a high pH level (which helps nicotine enter the blood stream faster), and a high portion of unprotonated (free base) nicotine.

It has been suggested by *The Economist* magazine that the ban on smoking tobacco indoors in some areas, such as Britain and New York City, may lead to a resurgence in the popularity of snuff as an alternative to tobacco smoking. Although the large-scale closure of British mines in the 1980s deprived the snuff industry of its major market since snuff became unfashionable (miners took snuff underground instead of smoking to avoid lethal explosions and fires), sales at Britain's largest snuff retailer have reportedly been rising at about 5% per year. Snuff is tobacco that you can snort

Chewing Tobacco

Chewing is one of the oldest ways of consuming tobacco leaves. Native Americans in both North and South America chewed the leaves of the plant, frequently mixed with lime. Modern chewing tobacco is produced in three forms: twist, plug, and scrap. A few manufacturers in the United Kingdom produce particularly strong twist tobacco meant for use in smoking pipes rather than chewing. These twists are not mixed with lime although they may be flavoured with whiskey, rum, cherry or other flavors common to pipe tobacco.

Twist is the oldest form. One to three high-quality leaves are braided and twisted into a rope while green, and then are cured in the same manner as other tobacco. Originally devised by sailors due to fire hazards of smoking at sea; and until recently this was done by farmers for their personal consumption in addition to other tobacco intended for sale. Modern twist is occasionally lightly sweetened. It is still sold commercially, but rarely seen outside of Appalachia. Popular brands are Mammoth Cave, Moore's Red Leaf, and Cumberland Gap. Users cut a piece off the twist and chew it, expectorating.

Plug chewing tobacco is made by pressing together cured tobacco leaves in a sweet (often molasses-based) syrup. Originally this was done by hand, but since the second half of the 19th century leaves were pressed between large tin sheets. The resulting sheet of tobacco is cut into plugs. Like twist, consumers sometimes cut, but more often bite off a piece of the plug to chew. Major brands are Days O Work and Cannonball.

Scrap, or looseleaf chewing tobacco, was originally the excess of plug manufacturing. It is sweetened like plug tobacco, but sold loose in bags rather than a plug. Looseleaf is one of the more popular forms of tobacco in modern times. Among those, popular brands are Red Man, Beechnut, Mail Pouch and Southern Pride. Looseleaf chewing tobacco can also be dipped. Of course, as far as people go, a person could prefer any type of chewing tobacco.

Snus

Swedish snus is different in that it is made from steam-cured tobacco, rather than fire-cured, and its health effects are markedly different, with epidemiological studies showing dramatically lower rates of cancer and other tobacco-related health problems than cigarettes, American "Chewing Tobacco", Indian Gutka or African varieties. Prominent Swedish brands are Swedish Match, Ettan, and Tree Ankare. In the Scandinavian countries, moist snuff comes either in loose powder form, to be pressed into a small ball or ovoid either by hand or with the use of a special tool. It is sometimes packaged in small bags, suitable for placing inside the upper lip, called "portion snuff".

In the United States, the Skoal brand of moist snuff distributes a similar product, packed with standard American moist snuff, often flavoured with fruits or liquors; these small bags are called "Skoal Bandits." These small bags keep the loose tobacco from becoming lodged between the user's teeth; they also generate less spittle when in contact with mucous membranes inside the mouth which extends the usage time of the tobacco product.

Since it is not smoked, snuff in general generates less of the nitrosamines and other carcinogens in the tar that forms from the partially anaerobic reactions in the smoldering smoked tobacco. The steam curing of snus rather than fire-curing or flue-curing of other smokeless tobaccos has been demonstrated to generate even fewer of such compounds than other varieties of snuff; 2.8 parts per mil for *Ettan* brand compared to as high as 127.9 parts per mil in American brands, according to a study by the State of Massachusetts Health Department.

It is hypothesized that the widespread use of snus by Swedish men (estimated at 30% of Swedish men, possibly because it is much cheaper than cigarettes), displacing tobacco smoking and other varieties of snuff, is responsible for the incidence of tobacco-related mortality in men being significantly lower in Sweden than any other European country. In contrast, since women are much less likely to use snus, their rate of tobacco-related deaths in Sweden is similar to that in other European countries. Snus is clearly less harmful than other tobacco products; according to Kenneth Warner, director of the University of Michigan Tobacco Research Network,

"The Swedish government has studied this stuff to death, and to date, there is no compelling evidence that it has any adverse health consequences. ... Whatever they eventually find out, it is dramatically less dangerous than smoking."

Public health researchers maintain that, nevertheless, even the low nitrosamine levels in snus cannot be completely risk free, but snus proponents maintain that inasmuch as snus is used as a substitute for smoking or a means to quit smoking, the net overall effect is positive, similar to the effect of nicotine patches, for instance. Snus is banned in the European Union countries outside of Sweden (regular snus, not portion, is allowed in Denmark and snus is also becoming a regular among Norwegians, as cigarettes are seen by Norwegian popular culture as untrendy and much more unhealthy than snus). Although this is officially for health reasons, it is widely regarded, in fact, as being for economic reasons, since other smokeless tobacco products (mainly from India) associated with much greater risk to health are sold too.

Although it lacks the carcinogenicity of high levels of nitrosamines, however, any harmful effects of nicotine will still be seen with snus usage. Current research concentrates on nicotine's effect on the circulatory system and on the pancreas.

On June 11, 2006, Reynolds Tobacco announced that it would be test marketing Camel brand snus in Portland, Oregon and Austin, Texas by the end of the month. The product would be manufactured in Sweden, in conjunction with British American Tobacco, manufacturers of BAT snus.

Creamy Snuff

Creamy snuff is a tobacco paste, consisting of tobacco, clove oil, glycerin, spearmint, menthol, and camphor, and sold in a toothpaste tube. It is marketed mainly to women in India, and is known by the brand names Ipco (made by Asha Industries), Denobac, Tona, Ganesh. It is locally known as "mishri" in some parts of Maharashtra. According to the U.S NIH-sponsored 2002 Smokeless Tobacco Fact Sheet, it is marketed as a dentifrice. The same factsheet also mentions that it is "often used to clean teeth". The manufacturer recommends letting the paste linger in the mouth before rinsing.

Tobacco Water

Tobacco water is a traditional organic insecticide used in domestic gardening. Tobacco dust can be used similarly.

It is produced by boiling strong tobacco in water, or by steeping the tobacco in water for a longer period. When cooled the mixture can be applied as a spray, or 'painted' on to the leaves of garden plants, where it will prove deadly to insects.

Basque *angulero* fishermen kill immature eels (elvers) in an infusion of tobacco leaves before parboiling them in salty water for transportation to market as *angulas*, a seasonal delicacy. .

Campaigns

There have been many campaigners against the growth of tobacco. New Zealand companies Reuben and Co. and Joseph's Nachos continue to protest against the growth and sale of tobacco throughout the world. Other well known protesters include Lance Tollenaar and Tim Smith, as well as the company owners, Joseph Griffiths and Reuben Palmer.

Sugarcane

Sugarcane or Sugar cane (*Saccharum*) is a genus of 6 to 37 species (depending on taxonomic interpretation) of tall grasses (family Poaceae, tribe Andropogoneae), native to warm temperate to tropical regions of the Old World. They have stout, jointed, fibrous stalks that are rich in sugar and measure 2 to 6 meters tall. All of the sugarcane species interbreed, and the major commercial cultivars are complex hybrids.

Cultivation and Uses

About 200 countries grow the crop to produce 1,324 million tons (more than six times the amount of sugar beet produced). As of the year 2005, the world's largest producer of sugar cane by far is Brazil. Uses of sugar cane include the production of sugar, Falernum, molasses, rum, cachaça (the national spirit of Brazil) and ethanol for fuel. The bagasse that remains after sugarcane crushing is used to provide both heat energy, used in the mill, and electricity, which is typically on-sold to the consumer electricity grid.

History

Sugarcane was originally from tropical Southeast Asia. Different species likely originated in different locations with

S. barberi originating in India and *S. edule* and *S. officinarum* coming from New Guinea. The thick stalk stores energy as sucrose in the sap. From this juice, sugar is extracted by evaporating the water. Crystallized sugar was reported 2500 years ago in India. Around the eighth century A.D., Arabs introduced sugar to the Mediterranean and it was cultivated in Spain. It was among the early crops brought to the Americas by Spaniards.

Sugarcane was, and is still is, extensively grown in the Caribbean, where it was first brought by Christopher Columbus during his second voyage to The Americas, initially to the island of Hispaniola. In colonial times, sugar was a major product of the triangular trade of New World raw materials, European manufactures, and African slaves. France found its sugarcane islands so valuable it effectively traded Canada to Britain for their return of Guadeloupe, Martinique and St. Lucia at the end of the Seven Years' War.

The Dutch similarly kept Suriname, a sugar colony in South America, instead of seeking the return of the New Netherlands (New Amsterdam). Cuban sugarcane produced sugar that received price supports from and a guaranteed market in the USSR; the dissolution of that country forced the closure of most of Cuba's sugar industry. Sugarcane remains an important part of the economy of Belize, Barbados, the Dominican Republic, Guadeloupe, Jamaica, Grenada, and other islands. The sugarcane industry is a major export for the Caribbean, but it is expected to collapse with the removal of European preferences by 2009.

Sugarcane production greatly influenced many tropical Pacific islands, most particularly Hawaii and Fiji. In these islands, sugar came to dominate the economic and political landscape after the indigenous societies had been invaded by Europeans and Americans, who promoted immigration from various Asian countries for workers to tend and harvest the crop. Sugar-industry policies eventually established the ethnic makeup of the island populations that now exist, profoundly affecting modern politics and society in the islands.

Brazil is a major grower of sugarcane, which is used to produce sugar and provide the ethanol used in making gasoline-ethanol blends (gasohol) for transportation fuel.

Cultivation

Sugarcane cultivation requires a tropical or subtropical climate, with a minimum of 600 mm (24 in) of annual moisture. It is one of the most efficient photosynthesizers in the plant kingdom, able to convert up to 2 percent of incident solar energy into biomass. In prime growing regions, such as Hawaii, sugarcane can produce 20 kg for each square meter exposed to the sun.

Sugarcane is propagated from cuttings, rather than from seeds; although certain types still produce seeds, modern methods of stem cuttings have become the most common method of reproduction. Each cutting must contain at least one bud, and the cuttings are usually planted by hand. Once planted, a stand of cane can be harvested several times; after each harvest, the cane sends up new stalks, called ratoons. Usually, each successive harvest gives a smaller yield, and eventually the declining yields justify replanting. Depending on agricultural practice, two to ten harvests may be possible between plantings.

Sugarcane is harvested by hand or mechanically. Hand harvesting accounts for more than half of the world's production, and is especially dominant in the developing world. When harvested by hand, the field is first set on fire. The fire spreads rapidly, burning away dry dead leaves, and killing any venomous snakes hiding in the crop, but leaving the water-rich stalks and roots unharmed. With knives (usually Cane Knives, but Machetes are also commonly used), harvesters then cut the standing cane just above the ground. A skilled harvester can cut 500 kg of sugarcane in an hour.

With mechanical harvesting, a sugarcane combine (or chopper harvester), a harvesting machine originally developed in Australia, is used. The machine cuts the cane at the base of the stalk, separates the cane from its leaves, and deposits the cane into a cart while blowing the cut leaves back onto the field. Such machines can harvest 30 tonnes of cane each hour, but cane harvested using these machines must be transported to the processing plant rapidly; once cut, sugarcane begins to lose its sugar content, and damage inflicted on the cane during mechanical harvesting accelerates this decay.

Pests

The most important sugarcane pests are the larvae of some lepidoptera species, including turnip moth, the sugarcane borer, *Diatraea saccharalis* and the Mexican rice borer (*Eoreuma loftini*), leaf-cutting ants, termites, spittlebugs (especially *Mahanarva fimbriolata* and *Deois flavopicta*) and the beetle *Migdolus fryanus*, among others.

Diseases

Processing

Traditionally, sugarcane has been processed in two stages. Sugarcane mills, located in sugarcane-producing regions, extract sugar from freshly harvested sugarcane, resulting in raw sugar for later refining, and in "mill white" sugar for local consumption. Sugar refineries, often located in heavy sugar-consuming regions, such as North America, Europe, and Japan, then purify raw sugar to produce refined white sugar, a product that is more than 99 percent pure sucrose. These two stages are slowly becoming blurred. Increasing affluence in the sugar-producing tropics has led to an increase in demand for refined sugar products in those areas, where a trend toward combined milling and refining has developed.

Milling

In a sugar mill, sugarcane is washed, chopped, and shredded by revolving knives. The shredded cane is repeatedly mixed with water and crushed between rollers; the collected juices (called garapa in Brazil) contain 10–15 percent sucrose, and the remaining fibrous solids, called bagasse, are burned for fuel. Bagasse makes a sugar mill more than self-sufficient in energy; the surplus bagasse can be used for animal feed, in paper manufacture, or burned to generate electricity for the local power grid.

The cane juice is next mixed with lime to adjust its pH to 7. This mixing arrests sucrose's decay into glucose and fructose, and precipitates out some impurities. The mixture then sits, allowing the lime and other suspended solids to settle out, and the clarified juice is concentrated in a multiple-effect evaporator to make a syrup about 60 percent by weight in sucrose.

This syrup is further concentrated under vacuum until it becomes supersaturated, and then seeded with crystalline sugar. Upon cooling, sugar crystallizes out of the syrup. A centrifuge is used to separate the sugar from the remaining liquid, or molasses. Additional crystallizations may be performed to extract more sugar from the molasses; the molasses remaining after no more sugar can be extracted from it in a cost-effective fashion is called blackstrap.

Raw sugar has a yellow to brown colour. If a white product is desired, sulphur dioxide may be bubbled through the cane juice before evaporation; this chemical bleaches many colour-forming impurities into colourless ones. Sugar bleached white by this *sulfitation* process is called "mill white," "plantation white," and "crystal sugar." This form of sugar is the form most commonly consumed in sugarcane-producing countries.

Refining

In sugar refining, raw sugar is further purified. It is first mixed with heavy syrup and then centrifuged clean. This process is called "affination"; its purpose is to wash away the outer coating of the raw sugar crystals, which is less pure than the crystal interior. The remaining sugar is then dissolved to make a syrup, about 70 percent by weight solids.

The sugar solution is clarified by the addition of phosphoric acid and calcium hydroxide, which combine to precipitate calcium phosphate. The calcium phosphate particles entrap some impurities and absorb others, and then float to the top of the tank, where they can be skimmed off. An alternative to this "phosphatation" technique is "carbonatation," which is similar, but uses carbon dioxide and calcium hydroxide to produce a calcium carbonate precipitate.

After any remaining solids are filtered out, the clarified syrup is decolorized by filtration through a bed of activated carbon; bone char was traditionally used in this role, but its use is no longer common. Some remaining colour-forming impurities adsorb to the carbon bed.

The purified syrup is then concentrated to supersaturation and repeatedly crystallized under vacuum, to produce white refined sugar. As in a sugar mill, the sugar crystals are separated from the molasses by centrifugation. Additional sugar is recovered by blending the remaining syrup with the washings from affination and again crystallizing to produce brown sugar. When no more sugar can be economically recovered, the final molasses still contains 20–30 percent sucrose and 15–25 percent glucose and fructose.

To produce granulated sugar, in which the individual sugar grains do not clump together, sugar must be dried. Drying is accomplished first by drying the sugar in a hot rotary dryer, and then by conditioning the sugar by blowing cool air through it for several days.

Ribbon Cane Syrup

Ribbon cane is a subtropical type that was once widely grown in southern United States, as far north as coastal North Carolina. The juice was extracted with horse or mule-powered crushers; the juice was boiled, like maple syrup, in a flat pan, and then used in the syrup to form as a sweetener for other foods. It is not a commercial crop nowadays, but a few growers try to keep alive the old traditions and find ready sales for their product. Most sugarcane production in the United States occurs in Florida and Louisiana, and to a lesser extent in Hawaii and Texas.

Sugarcane as Food

In most countries where sugarcane is cultivated, there are several foods and popular dishes derived from it, such as:

- Direct consumption of raw sugarcane cylinders or cubes, which are chewed to extract the juice, and the bagasse is spat out

- Freshly extracted juice (garapa, *guarab, guarapa, guarapo, papelón,* or *caldo de cana*) by hand or electrically operated small mills, with a touch of lemon and ice, makes a delicious and popular drink.
- Molasses, used as a sweetener and as a syrup accompanying other foods, such as cheese or cookies
- Rapadura, a candy made of flavoured solid brown sugar in Brazil, which can be consumed in small hard blocks, or in pulverized form (flour), as an add-on to other desserts.
- Sugarcane is also used in rum production, especially in the Caribbean.

Propagation-Fruit Plants

In case of fruits like Pomelo, Limes, etc. they bear fruits in 3 to 4 years, Litchi and mango take six to eight years before a bumper crop can be gathered. The plants raised by vegetative propagation will come to flowering and fruiting much earlier than the one obtained from seed. They might bear at the very first year after planting, but precocious bearing should not be encouraged. It will hamper the vigour of the fruit tree. Where seedlings are planted, the fruiting period is protracted and one is never certain of obtaining a good type from a seedling unless careful selection has been practised. Plants propagated by vegetative means retain the good qualities of their mother without any deterioration.

For instance, a seedling Kaghzi lime of a thin skinned mother, may have a thick rind and little juice while one propagated by gooties will perpetuate the thin skin character. Always buy from a reliable source as foliage differences cannot be depended on for judging the quality and type of the plant. Because to discover after eight years that a Langra Mango tree bears small acid fruits will be no recompense from having purchased the graft a few paisa cheaper from an unauthentic source.

Major Fruits

- *Banana (Musa paradisiaca)*: For vegetative propagation sucker is the most popular planting material. Among the suckers which arise from the rhizome, the sword suckers (having narrow sword-shaped leaves) are better than the water suckers (with broad leaves) and should be used.

- *Cashew (Anacardium occidentale):* The plants are propagated by seeds, air-layering, inarching and side grafting.
- *Oranges:* Oranges in India can be mainly divided into two groups—Sweet oranges (*Citrus sinensis*) The typical examples of sweet oranges in our country are Malta, Mosambi, Sathgudi and Washington Navel, etc., and of Mandarine group are all types of loose skinned oranges commonly known as Nagpur Santra, Assam Santra, Coorg Santra and Sikkim orange etc. Unlike the Mandarine orange, sweet oranges are tight skinned and heavy.

Sweet Oranges: Sweet oranges are usually propagated by budding.

Mandarine Oranges (C. reticulata): Budding on rough lemon and seed propagation is better prevalent in Santra oranges.

- *Lime (C. aurantifolia):* Seed propagation and budding are usually practised in sour lime. Sweet lime is propagated both by stem cutting and seed.
- *Shaddock (C. decumana):* Plants should be grown from gooties or buddlings.
- *Custard apple (Anona squoamosa):* Seedlings vary appreciably in their characters. Grafting by budding and inarching are usually characters. Grafting by budding and inarching are usually done on Bullock's Heart (*Anona reticulata*) plants, which is an allied species.
- *Grape (Vitis vinigera):* The grapes are usually propagated by stem cuttings. Seed propagation is used fro breeding purposes.
- *Guava (Psidium guajava):* It is propagated by seed as well as by air-layering, ground layering and inarching.
- *Jack fruit (Artocarpus integrifolia):* It is propagated by seed and inarching.

- *Litchi (Litchi chinensis):* Air layering is the usual method of propagation. Ground layering, budding, grafting and inarching are also practised. Plants, which are propagated by gooties, bear fruits in 4-5 years.
- *Mango (Mangifera indica):* Mango can be propagated by seed and by vegetative means such as budding, grafting, inarching, etc. Vegetatively propagated plants usually give good quality fruits. They also bear much earlier than the seed propagated plants.
- *Papaya (Carica papaya):* Papaya is propagated by seed, which should be sown at the early monsoon. Seedlings of 30 to 45 days age are 20-30 cms. Height should be transplanted in monsoon 2.5 to 4 metres apart.
- *Pineapple (Ananas comosus):* Pineapple grows from suckers, stumps, side shoots or crowns, but is usually propagated from slips and suckers. Pineapple suckers will give fruit a year ahead of plants raised from fruit crowns.
- *Bael (Aegle marmelos):* The plants are usually propagated by seed. Seedlings bear in 6-8 years but give best result after the 10th year.
- *Ber (Zizyphus jujuba):* It is usually seed propagated but shield and ring budding are also common.
- *Loquat (Eribotrya japonica):* The plants are propagated by gooties, which bear in 2-4 years. Seedlings take about 8 to 10 years to fruit.
- *Pomegranate (Punica granatum):* Plants raised through cuttings or gooties bear in 3 years while seedlings take 6-8 years and are never to be depended on.
- *Sapota (Achras sapota):* Ground layering, air layering and inarching are the usual methods of propagation.

Propagation of Ornamental Plants

Plants usually reproduce in two ways:

1. By seeds and
2. By vegetative parts of plant.

The letter method is very popular in the multiplication of fruit and ornamental plants.

Sexual Propagation or Propagation by Seeds: This is the easiest method of propagation of plants. In this method the seeds are sown, covered with a layer of soil or leaf mould and watered. After germination the seedlings are allowed to grow up to 4-leaf stage and then they are transplanted in the beds or pots. In some cases the seeds are directly sown in the ground. These seeds originate by the union of male and female gamete. During pollination pollens of male reproductive organ female reproductive organ. When the ovules are fertilized by the pollens of the same flower the process is known as self-pollination. Cross-pollination occurs when the pollens come from a different source and usually the pollinating agents are wind or insects. Self-pollination occurs when the pollens come from a different source and usually the pollinating agents are wind or insects. Self-pollinated seeds are likely true to type or variety, but the cross-pollinated ones may not resemble the parents for all the character. After pollination, male gametes fertilize ovules resulting in the production of seed.

A Sexual or Vegetative Propagation: The following are the reasons for propagating plants vegetatively:

1. Many plants do not produce seeds under local condition or have lost the ability of production of viable seed. It is found in several cases that plants which readily root from cuttings do not produce seeds *e.g.*, *Acalypha*, *Eranthemum*.
2. Plants, which are cross-pollinated and have different varieties in cultivation, produce seeds of heterogeneous mixture. In such plants particular type can be maintained only by vegetative method or by careful crossbreeding with the same variety.
3. Double dahlias when grown from seeds show a wide range of colour and also a mixture single, and semi-double. Apple pear, peach, mango etc., do not grow true to type from seeds.
4. Vegetative method of propagation results in earlier flowering and fruiting than those raised from seeds. Vegetative part of a fruiting plant is mature to bear, while a seedling take few years before the shoots ripen to produce flowers and fruits. Seedlings of *Amherstia*

nobilis or *Brownea* ariza require 7-8 years to flower but a layer starts flowering in the second year.

5. Plants are also vegetatively propagated to increase their resistance or to develop immunity to particular disease or pest.
6. A well-rooted vegetative part of a plant can adapt more readily to new environment and has greater possibility to flower and fruit than a seedling.

Many parts of plant are capable of giving rise to new plants under natural condition.

Bulbs: Bulbs are underground-modified stem in which the central axis is much shortened and fleshy leaf scales are closely pressed. Amaryllis, Crinum, Hymenocallis, Hemerocallis and Haemanthus, are usually multiplied by bulbs which arise from the main bulb. Cooperanthes, Zephyranthes and tube rose are also manly grown from bulbs.

Corms: Gladiolus produces new corms and cormels on old ones, which are used for multiplication.

Rhizomes, tubers and fleshy roots. Rhizomes are defined as more or less cylindrical branches growing laterally or upward through the soil. Many ornamental plants such as *Calathea, Anthurium, Alocasia, Alpinia, Hedychium, Heliconia, Gloriosa, Canna* produce rhizomes or rhizomatours stem with buds on it which can be cut into pieces and each one will produce a new plant. Root tubers of dahlia are storage organs and shoots arise from stem attached to the tubers.

Runner: When a slender stem grows out of a crown and trails along the ground it is called a runner or stolon. Chlorophytum, Episcia send out stolons and produce young plants from the nodes. It is then detached and grown separately.

Offsets: Many ornamental plants are propagated by this method. Sanseviera and *Agave americana* send out branches terminating in rosette of leaves which ultimately grow as new plants. These can be separated from the mother plants. Chrysanthemums also produce offsets, which are detached for multiplication of plants. Gerbera also sends out suckers on offsets.

Root Suckers: There are some plants, which produce suckers from roots and are detached from the mother plants for multiplication. *Millingtonia hortensis, Clerodendron splendens, Quisqualis indica* are few examples.

Trees: Most of the species of trees; grown in tropical conditions are raised from seeds. The seedlings with taproot grow tall and large and give necessary support against storm. Some species, however, often fail or produce seeds irregularly.

Seed: Species of *Cassia and Poinciana regia, Thespesia populnea, Peltophorum ferrugineum, couroupita guinensis, Acacia auriculi formis, Pithecolobium saman, Saraca indica, Spathodia campanulata, Lagerstroemia flos-regineae* and many other flowering trees produce seeds freely which germinate in seed compost consisting of garden soil and leafmould, one part each in bed or in seed pans. Seeds or mahogany have spongy seed coat and rot in excess moisture. Seeds of *Polyalthia* do not germinated if they become too dry. Seedlings of *Eucalyptus* and *Jacaranda* grow well in less humidity and temperature and should be sown in the spring.

Cutting: Plumerias root easily from stem cuttings. Cuttings are made in spring as excessive moisture in soil causes rotting. These are planted in sandy soil and light watering is done after callus formation. Plumerias produce large fruits containing many seeds but the seedlings do not flower before four years. Cutting from mature terminal shoot start flowering within few months. *Gliricidia* are also propagated from cuttings. In the case of *Spathodia campanulata* in addition to seed propagation, root suckers are also used.

Air layer and ground layer. *Gustavia augusta, Brownea ariza and B. grandiceps* though produce few fruits every year but the seedlings are very slow growing and are also propagated by air or ground layering. *Ficus elastica and Ficus krishnae* and *F.benjamina* are easily propagated from air layer.

Shrubs

Seeds: Few species of shrubs which produce seeds and the seedlings flower in one or two years without changing the character, are raised from seeds *e.g., Galphimia gracilis, Cassia* *glauca, Cassia didymobotrya, Solanum macranthum, Tecoma stans, Sophora tomentosa, Brya ebenus, Callindra speciosa Bauhinia acuminata, B. tomentosa and Caesalpinia pulcherrima speciosa, Ochna wightiana, O. squarrosa, Carissa carundas, Jacquinia ruscifolia, Bauhinia galpinii, Portlandia grandiflora* and *Calliandra speciosa* do not root easily from cutting and layering and so seed multiplication is commonly practised.

All species and varieties of *Acalypha, Angelonia, Aralia, Asystasia, Buddleia, Cestrum, Daedalacanthus, Eranthemum, Graprophyllum, Justicia, Lagerstroemia indica, Malvaviscus, Pentas, Poinsettia, Russelia, Jasminum sambc, Brugmansia, Stachytarpheta and Thunbergia are very easily propagated from cuttings.* In *Aralia, Eranthemum, Pentas, Aphelandra* and *Daedalacanthus*, tip cuttings produce quicker and better roots.

Green House Plants: Greenhouse plants thrive in shade and grow well in high humidity especially during the hot months. These are mostly grown for beautiful foliage though flowering plants like *Achimines* and *Pelargonium* need suitable protection during dry and hot season.

Seeds: Plants can be raised from seeds of *Coleus* but to maintain a particular variety vegetative propagation has to be done.

Stem Cutting: All the different species and varieties of *Aglaonema, Philodendron, Anthurium, Scindapsus, Monstera* and *Dieffenbachia,* have succulent stem which are cut into small pieces keeping one node in each and planted in ground or pot. The cuttings are planted horizontally about 1-2cm below the soil with the bud pointing upward. Several species of *Dracaena e.g., Dracaena ugandense, D. victoria, D. deremensis* "Bausii" D. *reflexa* "Variegata" are grown from top cuttings. The erect stem can also be cut into pieces with few nodes in each cutting and planted in soil. Top cuttings produce well-shaped plants after root formation, while shoots from lower cuttings have slower growth. *Episcia, Syngonium, Gynura, Fittonia, Pellionia, Coleus, Zebrina Pendula, Setcrasea Purpurea, Perperomia, Pillea and Strobilanthes dyerianus* are propagated from stem cuttings. It is safe to plant these soft cuttings in sand only. After root formation it can be transferred in pot or ground. Foliage begonias and African violets can be propagated from leaf cuttings but division is a safe method under our climatic conditions.

Species of ferns, *e.g.*, *Nephrolepis, Pteris, Ptyrogramma, Polypodium* and *Davallia* are divided with crown and rhizome. All palms produce seeds in suitable climate after attaining maturity. *Pritchardia, Caryota, Livistonia* and *Oreodoxa* often for seeds in Calcutta.

Propagation-Bulbs, Tubers

The bulbous plants are divided into two categories *i.e.*, hardy and tender bulbs. The hardy types can be left in the ground and are separated after 2-3 years for their multiplication (*e.g.* Amaryllis, tuberose, canna, zephyranthes, crinum, etc.). On the contrary, the tender types cannot be left in the ground after flowering and are to be lifted from the ground on maturity. After their treatment against diseases, these are to be stored in cold storage or cool places during off season for next year planting *e.g.* Gladiolus, Narcissus, Daffodils, Freesia, Dahlia, etc.

Propagation: The following are the common methods employed for propagation of bulbous plants;

i. *Off-sets, Cormlets or Bulblets:* Mother bulbs produce many bulblets, which are separated and planted for raising new crop. The intensity of bulblet production is a varietal character. Some varieties are very prolific bulblet producer whereas some produce sparse bulblets. It takes about 1-2 years for growing a bulblet into a full bulb.

ii. *Division:* It is followed in tubers, rhizomes and corms, which are divided carefully (in such a way that each piece contains at least one vegetative bud) and planted in the soil.

iii. *Terminal Cuttings:* These cuttings are mostly employed to propagate Dahlia and Rex begonia.

iv. *Seed:* This method is employed by the breeders to create new varieties *e.g.* Gladiolus, Dahlia, Freesia, Amaryllis, Lilies, etc.

Lifting of Bulbs and their Storage

Tender bulbs like Gladiolus, Dahlia, Narcissus, Daffodils, etc. are to be dug from the soil 10-12 weeks after flowering has been finished. Before lifting the bulbs, water is withheld. After digging, bulds are dried in shade for few days. Then these are treated with 0.2% Bavistin solution for 30 minutes and thereafter stored. Hardy bulbs are separated after 2-3 years and are again planted in the planting season.

Begonia sp. (Begoniaceae)

Begonias are grouped into three main classes according to root types *i.e.* rhizomatous (*Begonia red*), tuberous (*B. tuberhybrida*) and fibrous (*B. semperflorens*). Out of three types rhizomatous and fibrous rooted are grown in the plains whereas tuberous rooted can be grown successfully in hills. The important varieties of rhizomatous begonia are: Peace Majesty Silver Queen, Emperor Mikado, Can Can, Crimson Glory, Black Knight, Curly Star Dust, Dew Drop etc. The important varieties of fibrous rooted are: Goldilock, Bo-peep Little Gem, Ballet, Lady Frances, Pink Jewel, Flamengo, Cindrella, Charm, Silver Star, Pink Camellia etc. The tuberous rooted begonias are valued for their attractive flowers and are grouped into Rose form, Camellia flowered, Carnation flowered, Daffodil flowered or Picotee.

Canna Indica (Cannaceae)

Canna is a rhizomatous plant and is very easily propagated by dividing the rhizomes into 10-15 cm pieces during end of June.

Dahlia: Dahlia Variables (Compositae)

Propagation of dahlia is done by seeds, division of tubers and terminal cuttings. The propagation through seeds is easy and the best way to achieve striking mixtures of colourful flowers which are sown in September-October. The varieties which are being marketed in India are Giant Exhibition mixed, Dwarf Double Red Skin, Coltners hybrids, and Border Jewels, Rigoletto, and Citation. Tubers are stored during summer in cool place or in refrigerator. After careful separation, tubers

are planted directly in field in August. The care with a vegetative bud. The terminal cutting should be solid and made in September-October from plants and after treatment with seradix-I are planted in sand. It takes about 2-3 weeks for rooting and after that they are transplanted inpots (25-30cm) or in beds.

Vegetables

Most seeds normally remain viable for 2 or 3 years if stored under good conditions. To grow best vegetables either for home garden or for growing commercially try only certified seeds with, trueness to type and freedom from certain diseases. Good seeds are clean, viable, free from disease and true to the name variety. Therefore, buy only from seed firm of known integrity. High yielding, high price seeds should have 90% germination. Seeds of 50% germination is very poor.

Germination of Seeds: For germination of seeds adequate moisture, temperature and aeration are essential. The requirement of temperature for various vegetable seeds varies markedly. Some seeds do not germinate at low temperature while some others at high. Usually germination is optimum in between 40^0 F and 60^0 F. Seeds absorb moisture and swell and vital activities starts. Respiration begins and energy is supplied and this requires oxygen. Aeration is essential to supply oxygen. If supply of water is more or over wet aeration is poor and may hinder in germination.

Seed Treatments: Vegetable seeds are usually grown in nursery beds or in boxes. There are three types of seed treatments to control diseases.

1. Disinfestation
2. Disinfection.
3. Seed protection.

The first eliminates organisms present on the surface of seeds. Calcium hypochlorite, mercuric chloride and bromide water may be used. The second disinfectant eliminates organisms present within the seeds. For this hot water, formaldehyde and mercuric chloride are effective. In hot water treatment dry seeds are immersed in hot water 45 to 55^0 C for

10 to 15 minutes. The third treatment protectants are fungicides to protect seeds from soil fungi. Nursery soil should be drenched before sowing of seeds. Commercial materials are also now available to treat seeds like Captan, Cerason, Thiram, Bavistin, Agrosan GN and antibiotics such as Agrimycin (0.01%), Streptocyline (0.01%) etc. To secure healthy seedling the seed treatments should be invariably done. If the outside nursery bed contain worms, maggot and such insects a combination of insecticides and fungicides should be applied like Aldrin, Dieldrin with Captan, Thiram etc. All chemicals should be handled carefully according to directions of the manufacturer.

If boxes are used for growing seedling the soil should be disinfected by heating the soil to 180 F for atleast one hour. If nursery beds are used the soil may be disinfected by 40% Formalin. One part formaldehyde (40%) mixed in 50 parts of water and saturates the soil. After 24 hours of treatments the seeds may be sown. If captan and formaldehyde is used, the nursery soil may be drenched about 10-12 days before seed sowing.

Preparation of Nursery Beds: The nursery beds should be prepared before the soil treatments. The nursery beds should be of one meter width and length four to five meter. The soil should be cultivated to a find tilth. All weeds, stones etc. should be removed. The beds should be raised to 15 to 20 cm. heights. If necessary, shade or shelter may be provided. Usually total bed area of 80-100 sq.m. is sufficient for most of transplanted seedlings to cover one hectare.

NPK nursery mixture may be applied along with compost on FYM during preparation of soil. After complete preparation and levelling the beds should he given soil treatment as mentioned above.

Sowing of Seeds

The vegetable seeds should be sown in nursery beds in lines at 1.5-2 cm. below surface soiled at a distance of 5-6 cm. The distance from line to line should be 10-15 cm. After sowing cover the seeds with sieved compost very lightly. The beds should be watered with a sprinkler. The above distance from plant to plant or row to row may be changed according to size of seeds, kind of vegetables and type of seedlings. Similarly the depth of covering with compost varies with the kind of seed. Very fine seeds may be dusted over the nursery bed. Covering of other seeds may be one to two times their minimum diameter. During germination and after sprinkle water in the beds but no excessive. Over watering creates high humidity and poor aeration and contributes to "damping off" disease.

To transplant the vegetable seedlings to its permanent location the seedlings should be stocky, healthy and vigorous rather than spindly, weak and elongated plants. Moderate temperatures produce stocky growth. To harden some vegetable seedlings, seedlings may be transplanted one or two times to another nursery bed. In large scale condition watering may be withheld two to three days ahead of transplanting to permanent site.

The young seedlings in the nursery bed should protected against diseases and pests. Regular spray to young plants with Malathion 50 EC or Dithane M-45 or Sevin (0.2%) similar material at 10-15 days interval is necessary.

Most of the vegetable seedlings in the nursery bed is ready for transplanting when the seedlings are 4 to 6 weeks old. During uprooting every care should be taken not to damage roots. Light watering should be given at least 12 hours before lifting.

Spece Crops

Black Pepper

Black pepper (*Piper nigrum*) is a flowering vine in the family Piperaceae, cultivated for its fruit, which is usually dried and used as a spice and seasoning. The same fruit is also used to produce white pepper and green pepper. Black pepper is native to South India and is extensively cultivated there and elsewhere in tropical regions. The fruit, known as a **peppercorn** when dried, is a small drupe five millimetres in diameter, dark red when fully mature, containing a single seed.

Dried ground pepper is one of the most common spices in European cuisine and its descendants, having been known and prized since antiquity for both its flavour and its use as a medicine. The spiciness of black pepper is due to the chemical piperine. Ground black peppercorn, usually referred to simply as "pepper", may be found on nearly every dinner table in some parts of the world, often alongside table salt.

The word "pepper" is derived from the Sanskrit *pippali*, via the Latin *piper* and Old English *pipor*. The Latin word is also the source of German *pfeffer*, French *poivre*, Dutch *peper*, and other similar forms. In the 16th century, *pepper* started referring to the unrelated New World chile peppers as well. "Pepper" was used in a figurative sense to mean "spirit" or "energy" at least as far back as the 1840s; in the early 20th century, this was shortened to *pep*.

Varieties of Pepper

Black pepper is produced from the still-green unripe berries of the pepper plant. The berries are cooked briefly in hot water, both to clean them and to prepare them for drying. The heat ruptures cell walls in the fruit, speeding the work of browning enzymes during drying. The berries are dried in the sun or by machine for several days, during which the fruit around the seed shrinks and darkens into a thin, wrinkled black layer. Once dried, the fruits are called black peppercorns.

White pepper consists of the seed only, with the fruit removed. This is usually accomplished by allowing fully ripe berries to soak in water for about a week, during which the flesh of the fruit softens and decomposes. Rubbing then removes what remains of the fruit, and the naked seed is dried. Alternative processes are used for removing the outer fruit from the seed, including removal of the outer layer from black pepper produced from unripe berries.

In the U.S., white pepper is often used in dishes like light-coloured sauces or mashed potatoes, where ground black pepper would visibly stand out. There is disagreement regarding which is generally spicier. They do have differing flavours due to the presence of certain compounds in the outer fruit layer of the berry that are not found in the seed. Green pepper, like black, is made from the unripe berries. Dried green peppercorns are treated in a manner that retains the green colour, such as treatment with sulphur dioxide or freeze-drying. Pickled peppercorns, also green, are unripe berries preserved in brine or vinegar. Fresh, unpreserved green pepper berries, largely unknown in the West, are used in some Asian cuisines, particularly Thai cuisine. Their flavour has been described as piquant and fresh, with a bright aroma. They decay quickly if not dried or preserved.

A rarely seen product called pink pepper or red pepper consists of ripe red pepper berries preserved in brine and vinegar. Even more rarely seen, ripe red peppercorns can also be dried using the same colour-preserving techniques used to produce green pepper. Pink pepper from *Piper nigrum* is distinct from the more-common dried "pink peppercorns", which are the fruits of a plant from a different family, the Peruvian pepper tree, *Schinus molle*, and its relative the Brazilian pepper tree, *Schinus terebinthifolius*. In years past there was debate as to the health safety of pink peppercorns, which is mostly no longer an issue. Sichuan peppercorn is another "pepper" that is botanically unrelated to black pepper.

Peppercorns are often categorised under a label describing their region or port of origin. Two well-known types come from India's Malabar Coast: Malabar pepper and Tellicherry pepper. Tellicherry is a higher-grade pepper, made from the largest, ripest 10% of berries from Malabar plants grown on Mount Tellicherry. Sarawak pepper is produced in the Malaysian portion of Borneo, and Lampong pepper on Indonesia's island of Sumatra. White Muntok pepper is another Indonesian product, from Bangka Island.

The Pepper Plant

The pepper plant is a perennial woody vine growing to four metres in height on supporting trees, poles, or trellises. It is a spreading vine, rooting readily where trailing stems touch the ground. The leaves are alternate, entire, five to ten centimetres long and three to six centimetres broad. The flowers are small, produced on pendulous spikes four to eight centimetres long at the leaf nodes, the spikes lengthening to seven to 15 centimetres as the fruit matures.

Black pepper is grown in soil that is neither too dry nor susceptible to flooding, moist, well-drained and rich in organic matter. The plants are propagated by cuttings about 40 to 50 centimetres long, tied up to neighbouring trees or climbing frames at distances of about two metres apart; trees with rough bark are favoured over those with smooth bark, as the pepper plants climb rough bark more readily. Competing plants are cleared away, leaving only sufficient trees to provide shade and permit free ventilation. The roots are covered in leaf mulch and manure, and the shoots are trimmed twice a year. On dry soils the young plants require watering every other day during the dry season for the first three years. The plants bear fruit from the fourth or fifth year, and typically continue to bear fruit for seven years. The cuttings are usually cultivars, selected both for yield and quality of fruit.

A single stem will bear 20 to 30 fruiting spikes. The harvest begins as soon as one or two berries at the base of the spikes begin to turn red, and before the fruit is mature, but when full grown and still hard; if allowed to ripen, the berries lose pungency, and ultimately fall off and are lost. The spikes are collected and spread out to dry in the sun, then the peppercorns are stripped off the spikes.

History

Pepper has been used as a spice in India since prehistoric times. J. Innes Miller notes that while pepper was grown in southern Thailand and in Malaysia, its most important source was India, particularly the Malabar Coast, in what is now the state of Kerala. Peppercorns were a much prized trade good, often referred to as "black gold" and used as a form of commodity money. The term "peppercorn rent" still exists today.

The ancient history of black pepper is often interlinked with (and confused with) that of long pepper, the dried fruit of closely related *Piper longum*. The Romans knew of both and often referred to either as just "piper". In fact, it was not until the discovery of the New World and of chile peppers that the popularity of long pepper entirely declined. Chile peppers, some of which when dried are similar in shape and taste to long pepper, were easier to grow in a variety of locations more convenient to Europe.

Until well after the Middle Ages, virtually all of the black pepper found in Europe, the Middle East, and North Africa travelled there from India's Malabar region. By the 16th century, pepper was also being grown in Java, Sunda, Sumatra, Madagascar, Malaysia, and elsewhere in Southeast Asia, but these areas traded mainly with China, or used the pepper locally. Ports in the Malabar area also served as a stop-off point for much of the trade in other spices from farther east in the Indian Ocean.

Black pepper, along with other spices from India and lands farther east, changed the course of world history. It was in some part the preciousness of these spices that led to the European efforts to find a sea route to India and consequently to the European colonial occupation of that country, as well as the European discovery and colonization of the Americas.

Ancient Times

Black peppercorns were found lodged in the nostrils of Ramesses II, placed there as part of the mummification rituals shortly after his death in 1213 BCE. Little else is known about the use of pepper in ancient Egypt, nor how it reached the Nile from India.

Pepper (both long and black) was known in Greece at least as early as the 4th century BCE, though it was probably an uncommon and expensive item that only the very rich could afford. Trade routes of the time were by land, or in ships which hugged the coastlines of the Arabian Sea. Long pepper, growing in the northwestern part of India, was more accessible than the black pepper from further south; this trade advantage, plus long pepper's greater spiciness, probably made black pepper less popular at the time.

By the time of the early Roman Empire, especially after Rome's conquest of Egypt in 30 BCE, open-ocean crossing of the Arabian Sea directly to southern India's Malabar Coast was near routine. Details of this trading across the Indian Ocean have been passed down in the *Periplus of the Erythraean Sea*. According to the Roman geographer Strabo, the early Empire sent a fleet of around 120 ships on an annual one-year trip to India and back.

The fleet timed its travel across the Arabian Sea to take advantage of the predictable monsoon winds. Returning from India, the ships travelled up the Red Sea, from where the cargo was carried overland or via the Nile Canal to the Nile River, barged to Alexandria, and shipped from there to Italy and Rome. The rough geographical outlines of this same trade route would dominate the pepper trade into Europe for a millennium and a half to come.

With 'ships sailing directly to the Malabar coast, black pepper was now travelling a shorter trade route than long pepper, and the prices reflected it. Pliny the Elder's *Natural History* tells us the prices in Rome around 77 CE: "Long pepper is fifteen denarii per pound, while that of white pepper is seven, and of black, four." Pliny also complains "there is no year in which India does not drain the Roman Empire of fifty million sesterces," and further moralises on pepper:

It is quite surprising that the use of pepper has come so much into fashion, seeing that in other substances which we use, it is sometimes their sweetness, and sometimes their appearance that has attracted our notice; whereas, pepper has nothing in it that can plead as a recommendation to either fruit or berry, its only desirable quality being a certain pungency; and yet it is for this that we import it all the way from India! Who was the first to make trial of it as an article of food? and who, I wonder, was the man that was not content to prepare himself by hunger only for the satisfying of a greedy appetite? (*N.H.* 12.14)

Black pepper was a well-known and widespread, if expensive, seasoning in the Roman Empire. Apicius' De re coquinaria, a 3rd-century cookbook probably based at least partly on one from the 1st century CE, includes pepper in a majority of its recipes. Edward Gibbon wrote, in *The History of the Decline and Fall of the Roman Empire*, that pepper was "a favourite ingredient of the most expensive Roman cookery".

Postclassical Europe

Pepper was so valuable that it was often used as collateral or even currency. The taste for pepper (or the appreciation of its monetary value) was passed on to those who would see Rome fall. It is said that Alaric the Visigoth and Attila the Hun each demanded from Rome a ransom of more than a ton of pepper when they besieged the city in 5th century. After the fall of Rome, others took over the middle legs of the spice trade, first the Persians and then the Arabs; Innes Miller cites the account of Cosmas Indicopleustes, who travelled east to India, as proof that "pepper was still being exported from India in the sixth century". By the end of the Dark Ages, the central portions of the spice trade were firmly under Islamic control. Once into the Mediterranean, the trade was largely monopolised by Italian powers, especially Venice and Genoa. The rise of these city-states was funded in large part by the spice trade.

A riddle authored by Saint Aldhelm, a 7th-century Bishop of Sherborne, sheds some light on black pepper's role in England at that time:

I am black on the outside, clad in a wrinkled cover,

Yet within I bear a burning marrow.

I season delicacies, the banquets of kings, and the luxuries of the table,

Both the sauces and the tenderized meats of the kitchen.

But you will find in me no quality of any worth,

Unless your bowels have been rattled by my gleaming marrow.

It is commonly believed that during the Middle Ages, pepper was used to conceal the taste of partially rotten meat. There is no evidence to support this claim, and historians view it as highly unlikely: in the Middle Ages, pepper was a luxury item, affordable only to the wealthy, who certainly had unspoiled meat available as well. Similarly, the belief that pepper was widely used as a preservative is questionable: it is true that piperine, the compound that gives pepper its spiciness, has some antimicrobial properties, but at the concentrations present when pepper is used as a spice, the effect is small. Salt is a much more effective preservative, and salt-cured meats were common fare, especially in winter. However, pepper and other spices probably did play a role in improving the taste of long-preserved meats.

Its exorbitant price during the Middle Ages—and the monopoly on the trade held by Italy—was one of the inducements which led the Portuguese to seek a sea route to India. In 1498, Vasco da Gama became the first European to reach India by sea; asked by Arabs in Calicut (who spoke Spanish and Italian) why they had come, his representative replied, "we seek Christians and spices."

Though this first trip to India by way of the southern tip of Africa was only a modest success, the Portuguese quickly returned in greater numbers and used their superior naval firepower to eventually gain complete control of trade on the Arabian sea. This was the start of the first European empire in Asia, given additional legitimacy (at least from a European perspective) by the 1494 Treaty of Tordesillas, which granted Portugal exclusive rights to the half of the world where black pepper originated.

The Portuguese proved unable to maintain their stranglehold on the spice trade for long. The old Arab and Venetian trade networks successfully smuggled enormous quantities of spices through the patchy Portuguese blockade, and pepper once again flowed through Alexandria and Italy, as well as around Africa. In the 17th century, the Portuguese lost almost all of their valuable Indian Ocean possessions to the Dutch and the English. The pepper ports of Malabar fell to the Dutch in the period 1661–1663.

As pepper supplies into Europe increased, the price of pepper declined (though the total value of the import trade generally did not). Pepper, which in the early Middle Ages had been an item exclusively for the rich, started to become more of an everyday seasoning among those of more average means. Today, pepper accounts for one-fifth of the world's spice trade.

China

It is possible that black pepper was known in China in the 2nd century BCE, if poetic reports regarding an explorer named Tang Meng are correct. Sent by Emperor Wu to what is now southwest China, Tang Meng is said to have come across something called *jujiang* or "sauce-betel". He was told it came from the markets of Shu, an area in what is now the Sichuan province. The traditional view among historians is that "sauce-betel" is a sauce made from betel leaves, but arguments have been made that it actually refers to pepper, either long or black.

In the 3rd century CE, black pepper made its first definite appearance in Chinese texts, as *hujiao* or "foreign pepper". It does not appear to have been widely known at the time, failing to appear in a 4th-century work describing a wide variety of spices from beyond China's southern border, including long pepper. By the 12th century, however, black pepper had become a popular ingredient in the cuisine of the wealthy and powerful, sometimes taking the place of China's native Sichuan pepper (the tongue-numbing dried fruit of an unrelated plant).

Marco Polo testifies to pepper's popularity in 13th-century China when he relates what he is told of its consumption in the city of Kinsay (Zhejiang): "... Messer Marco heard it stated by one of the Great Kaan's officers of customs that the quantity of pepper introduced daily for consumption into the city of Kinsay amounted to 43 loads, each load being equal to 223 lbs." Marco Polo is not considered a very reliable source regarding China, and this second-hand data may be even more suspect, but if this estimated 10,000 pounds (4,500 kg) a day for one city is anywhere near the truth, China's pepper imports may have dwarfed Europe's.

Pepper as a Medicine

Like all eastern spices, pepper was historically both a seasoning and a medicine. Long pepper, being stronger, was often the preferred medication, but both were used.

Black peppercorns figure in remedies in Ayurveda, Siddha and Unani medicine in India. The 5th century *Syriac Book of Medicines* prescribes pepper (or perhaps long pepper) for such illnesses as constipation, diarrhea, earache, gangrene, heart disease, hernia, hoarseness, indigestion, insect bites, insomnia, joint pain, liver problems, lung disease, oral abscesses, sunburn, tooth decay, and toothaches. Various sources from the 5th century onward also recommend pepper to treat eye problems, often by applying salves or poultices made with pepper directly to the eye. There is no current medical evidence that any of these treatments has any benefit; pepper applied directly to the eye would be quite uncomfortable and possibly damaging.

Pepper has long been believed to cause sneezing; this is still believed true today. Some sources say that piperine irritates the nostrils, causing the sneezing; some say that it is just the effect of the fine dust in ground pepper, and some say that pepper is not in fact a very effective sneeze-producer at all. Few if any controlled studies have been carried out to answer the question.

Pepper is eliminated from the diet of patients having abdominal surgery and ulcers because of its irritating effect upon the intestines, being replaced by what is referred to as a bland diet.

Pepper is sometimes used to stop light bleeding in restaurant kitchens.

Flavour

Pepper gets its spicy heat mostly from the piperine compound, which is found both in the outer fruit and in the seed. Refined piperine, milligram-for-milligram, is about one per cent as hot as the capsaicin in chile peppers. The outer fruit layer, left on black pepper, also contains important odour-contributing terpenes including pinene, sabinene, limonene, caryophyllene, and linalool, which give citrusy, woody, and floral notes. These scents are mostly missing in white pepper, which is stripped of the fruit layer. White pepper can gain some different odours (including musty notes) from its longer fermentation stage.

Pepper loses flavour and aroma through evaporation, so airtight storage helps preserve pepper's original spiciness longer. Pepper can also lose flavour when exposed to light, which can transform piperine into nearly tasteless isochavicine. Once ground, pepper's aromatics can evaporate quickly; most culinary sources recommend grinding whole peppercorns immediately before use for this reason. Handheld pepper mills (or "pepper grinders"), which mechanically grind or crush whole peppercorns, are used for this, sometimes instead of pepper shakers, dispensers of pre-ground pepper. Spice mills such as pepper mills were found in European kitchens as early as the 14th century, but the mortar and pestle used earlier for crushing pepper remained a popular method for centuries after as well.

World Trade

Peppercorns are, by monetary value, the most widely traded spice in the world, accounting for 20 percent of all spice imports in 2002. The price of pepper can be volatile, and this figure fluctuates a great deal year to year; for example, pepper made up 39 percent of all spice imports in 1998. By weight, slightly more chile peppers are traded worldwide than peppercorns. The International Pepper Exchange is located in Kochi, India.

Vietnam has recently become the world's largest producer and exporter of pepper (85,000 long tons in 2003). Other major producers include Indonesia (67,000 tons), India (65,000 tons), Brazil (35,000 tons), Malaysia (22,000 tons), Sri Lanka (12,750 tons), Thailand, and China. Vietnam dominates the export market, using almost none of its production domestically. In 2003, Vietnam exported 82,000 tons of pepper, Indonesia 57,000 tons, Brazil 37,940 tons, Malaysia 18,500 tons, and India 17,200 tons.

Cardamom

The name **cardamom** (sometimes written **cardamon**) is used for heba within two genera of the ginger family Zingiberaceae, namely *Elettaria* and *Amomum*.

Types of Cardamom and their Distribution

The two main *genera* of the ginger family that are named as forms of cardamom are distributed as follows:

- *Elettaria* (commonly called cardamom, green cardamom, or true cardamom) is distributed from India to Malaysia.

- *Amomum* (commonly known as black cardamom, brown cardamom, Kravan, Java cardamom, Bengal cardamom, Siamese cardamom, white or red cardamom) is distributed mainly in Asia and Australia.

Uses

All the different cardamom species and varieties are used mainly as cooking spices and as medicines. In general,

- *Elettaria cardamomum* (the usual type of cardamom) is used as a spice, a masticatory, and in medicine; it is also sometimes smoked; it is used as a food plant by the larva of the moth *Endoclita hosei*.
- *Amomum* is used as an ingredient in traditional systems of medicine in China, India, Korea, Japan, and Vietnam.
- Can be used as a traditional flavouring to Turkish coffee.
- Is often used in the traditional Indian tea, or chai, especially with milk and sugar.

Uses in Cuisines Around the World

Cardamom has a strong, unique taste, with an intensely aromatic fragrance. It is a common ingredient in Indian cooking, and is often used in baking in Scandinavia. One of the most expensive spices by weight, little is needed to impart the flavour. Cardamom is best stored in pod form, because once the seeds are exposed or ground, they quickly lose their flavour. However, high-quality ground cardamom is often more readily (and cheaply) available, and is an acceptable substitute. For recipes requiring whole cardamom pods, a generally accepted equivalent is 10 pods equals 1½ teaspoons of ground cardamom.

In Traditional Medicine

In India, green cardamom (*A. subulatum*), or "elaichi," is broadly used to treat infections in teeth and gums, to prevent and treat throat troubles, congestion of the lungs and pulmonary tuberculosis, inflammation of eyelids and also digestive disorders. It is also reportedly used as an antidote for both snake and scorpion venom.

Species in the genus *Amomum* are also used in traditional Indian medicine. Among other species, varieties and cultivars,

Amomum villosum is used in traditional Chinese medicine to treat stomach-aches, constipation, dysentery, and other digestion problems. "Tsaoko" cardamom is cultivated in Yunnan, China, both for medicinal purposes and as a spice.

Ginger

Ginger is commonly used as a spice in cuisines throughout the world. Though commonly referred to as a root, it is actually the rhizome of the monocotyledonous perennial plant *Zingiber officinale*. Originating in southern China, cultivation of ginger spread to India, Southeast Asia, West Africa, and the Caribbean.

Chemistry

Ginger contains up to 3% of an essential oil that causes the fragrance of the spice. The main constituents are sesquiterpenoids with (-)-zingiberene as the main component. Lesser amounts of other sesquiterpenoids (a-sesquiphell-andrene, bisabolene and farnesene) and a small monoterpenoid fraction (a-phelladrene, cineol, and citral) have also been identified.

The pungent taste of ginger is due to nonvolatile phenylpropanoids (particularly gingerol and zingerone) and diarylheptanoids (gingeroles and shoagoles); the latter are more pungent and form from the former when ginger is dried. With a specific procedure is used for cooking, where ginger root acquires a soda form and transforms gingerol into zingerone, which is less pungent and has a spicy-sweet aroma.

Culinary Uses

Young ginger roots are juicy and fleshy with a very mild taste. They are often pickled in vinegar or sherry as a snack or just cooked as an ingredient in many dishes. They can also be stewed in boiling water to make ginger tea, to which honey is often added as a sweetener. Mature ginger roots are fibrous and nearly dry. The juice from old ginger roots is extremely potent and is often used as a spice in Chinese cuisine to flavour dishes such as in seafood and mutton.

Ginger is also candied, is used as a flavoring for candy, cookies, crackers and cake, and is the main flavour in ginger ale, a sweet, carbonated, non-alcoholic beverage, as well as the similar, but somewhat spicier beverage ginger beer. A ginger-flavoured liqueur called Canton is produced in the Guangdong province of China; it is advertised to be based on a recipe created for the rulers of the Qing Dynasty and made from six different varieties of ginger. Green ginger wine is a ginger flavoured wine produced in the United Kingdom by Crabbie's and Stone's and traditionally sold in a green glass bottle. Ginger is also used as a spice added to hot coffee and tea.

In Japan, ginger is pickled to make beni shoga and gari or grated and used raw on tofu or noodles.

In Western cuisine, ginger is traditionally restricted to sweet foods, such as ginger ale, gingerbread, ginger snaps, ginger cake and ginger biscuits.

Powdered dry ginger root (ground ginger) is typically used to add spiciness to gingerbread and other recipes. Ground and fresh ginger taste quite different and ground ginger is a particularly poor substitute for fresh ginger. Fresh ginger can be successfully substituted for ground ginger and should be done at a ratio of 6 parts fresh for 1 part ground. You generally achieve better results by substituting only half the ground ginger for fresh ginger.

In Myanmar, ginger is used in a salad dish called *gyin-tho*, which consists of shredded ginger preserved in oil, and a variety of nuts and seeds.

In traditional Korean Kimchi, ginger is minced finely and added into the ingredients of the spicy paste just before the fermenting process.

In India, ginger is used in all sub-varieties of the Indian cuisines. In south India, ginger is used in the production of a candy called Inji-murappa ("ginger candy" from Tamil). This candy is mostly sold by vendors to bus passengers in bus stops and in small tea shops as a locally produced item. Candied ginger is also very famous around these parts. Additionally, in Tamil Nadu, especially in the Tanjore belt, a variety of ginger which is less spicy is used when tender to make fresh pickle with the combination of lemon juice or vinegar, salt and tender green chillies. This kind of pickle was generally made before the invention of refrigeration and stored for a maximum of 4-5 days. The pickle gains a mature flavour when the juices cook the ginger over the first 24 hours. Ginger is used in the curries of North Indian food or cooked into the food.

In South East Asia, the flower of a type of ginger is used in cooking. This unopened flower is known in the Malay language as Bunga Kantan, and is used in salads and also as garnish for sour-savoury soups, like Assam Laksa.

Ginger has a sialagogue action, stimulating the production of saliva.

Medicinal Uses

One medical research study had results indicating that ginger might be an effective treatment for nausea caused by motion sickness or other illness, The study however, failed to show a significant difference between ginger and a placebo. There are several proposed mechanisms of action for the anti-emetic properties of ginger but there is not yet conclusive support for any particular model.

Modern research on nausea and motion sickness used approximately 1 gram of ginger powder daily. Though there are claims for efficacy in all causes of nausea, the PDR recommends against taking ginger root for morning sickness commonly associated with pregnancy due to possible mutagenic effects. Nevertheless, Chinese women traditionally have taken ginger root during pregnancy to combat morning sickness. The Natural Medicines Comprehensive Database (compiled by health professionals and pharmacists), states that ginger is likely safe for use in pregnancy when used orally in amounts found in foods. Ginger ale and ginger beer have been recommended as "stomach settlers" for generations in countries where the beverages are made. Ginger water was commonly used to avoid heat cramps in the United States in the past.

In Western-hemisphere nations, powdered dried ginger root is made into capsules and sold in pharmacies for medicinal use. In the US, ginger is not approved by the FDA for the treatment or cure of any disease. Ginger is instead sold as an unregulated dietary supplement. In India, ginger is applied as a paste to the temples to relieve headache. In Myanmar, ginger and local sweet (Htan nyat) which is made from palm tree juice are boiled together and taken to prevent the Flu. A hot ginger drink (made with sliced ginger cooked in sweetened water or a Coca-Cola-like drink) has been reported as a folk medicine for common cold.

Ginger has also historically been used in folk medicine to treat inflammation, although medical studies as to the efficacy of ginger in decreasing inflammation have shown mixed results. There are several studies that demonstrate a decrease in joint pain from arthritis after taking ginger, though the results have not been consistent from study to study. It may also have blood thinning and cholesterol lowering properties, making it theoretically effective in treating heart disease; while early studies have shown some efficacy, it is too early to determine whether further research will bear this out.

The medical form of ginger historically was called "Jamaica ginger"; it was classified as a stimulant and carminative, being much used for dyspepsia and colic. It was also frequently employed to disguise the taste of nauseous medicines. The tea brewed from this root was an old-fashioned remedy for colds.

The characteristic odour and flavour of ginger root is caused by a mixture of zingerone, shoagoles and gingerols, volatile oils that compose about 1%–3% by weight of fresh ginger. The gingerols have analgesic, sedative, antipyretic, antibacterial, and GI tract motility effects.

Ginger is on the GRAS list from FDA. However, like other herbs, ginger may be harmful because it may interact with other medications, such as warfarin; hence, a physician or pharmacist should be consulted before taking the herb. Ginger is also contraindicated in people suffering from gallstones, because the herb promotes the release of bile from the gallbladder.

Ginger Allergies

Some people are allergic to ginger. Generally, this is reported as having a gaseous component. This may take the form of flatulence, or it may take the form of an extreme constriction or tightening in the throat necessitating uncontrollable burping to relieve the pressure.

Horticulture

Ginger produces clusters of white and pink flower buds that bloom into yellow flowers. Because of the aesthetic appeal and the adaptivity of the plant to warm climates, ginger is often used as landscaping around subtropical homes. It is a perennial reed-like plant with annual leafy stems, three to four feet high.

Historical methods of gathering the root describes, when the stalk withers, it is immediately scalded, or washed and scraped, in order to kill it and prevent sprouting. The former method, applied generally to the older and poorer roots, produces Black Ginger; the latter, gives White Ginger. The natural colour of the "white" scraped ginger is a pale buff—it is often whitened by bleaching or liming, but generally at the expense of some of its real value.

References in popular culture:

- To members of the Race, an alien species in Harry Turtledove's best-selling novel series Worldwar, ginger is a highly addictive, psychoactive drug, with an effect similar to that of cocaine or PCP in humans.
- In Cockney rhyming slang, *ginger* is a derogatory euphemism for *homosexual*. The original slang rhymed *queer* with *ginger beer*.
- In the west of Scotland (particularly Glasgow), *ginger* is a term for any carbonated soft drink.
- Before the First World War, it was common for mounted regiments to receive large vats of root ginger before public ceremonies, which were peeled and cut into suppositories for the horses. The burning sensation made the horses hold their tails up; this practice is called Figging or feaguing.
- Ginger is also a common slang term in Great Britain for red-haired individuals, while In North America (USA and Canada) terms involving the word "carrot" are much

more common and in Australian English slang, a red-head is a *bluey / blooie*.

Similar Species

Myoga (*Zingiber mioga* Roscoe) appears in Japanese cuisine; the flower buds are the part eaten.

Another plant in the *Zingiberaceae* family, galangal, is used for similar purposes as ginger in Thai cuisine. Galangal is also called Thai ginger. Also referred to as galangal, fingerroot (*Boesenbergia rotunda*), or Chinese ginger or the Thai *krachai*, is used in cooking and medicine.

A dicotyledonous native species of eastern North America, *Asarum canadense*, is also known as "wild ginger", and its root has similar aromatic properties, but it is not related to true ginger and should not be used as a substitute because it contains the carcinogen aristolochic acid. This plant is also a powerful diuretic, or urinary stimulator. It is part of the Aristolochiaceae family.

Turmeric

Turmeric (*Curcuma longa*) is a member of the ginger family, Zingiberaceae. It's also called tumeric or kunyit in some Asian countries.

Its dried roots are ground into a deep yellow spice commonly used in curries and other South Asian cuisine. Its active ingredient is curcumin and it has an earthy, bitter, peppery flavour. Sangli, a town in the southern part of the Indian state of Maharashtra, is the largest and most important trading centre for turmeric in Asia or perhaps in the entire world.

Uses

Food: Turmeric has found application in canned beverages, baked products, dairy products, ice cream, yogurt, yellow cakes, biscuits, popcorn-colour, sweets, cake icings, cereals, sauces, gelatins, etc. It is a significant ingredient in most commercial curry powders.

Turmeric (coded as E100 when used as a food additive) is used to protect food products from sunlight. The oleoresin is used for oil-containing products. The curcumin/polysorbate solution or curcumin powder dissolved in alcohol is used for water containing products. Over-colouring, such as in pickles, relishes and mustard, is sometimes used to compensate for fading.

In combination with annatto (E160b), turmeric has been used to colour cheeses, dry mixes, salad dressings, winter butter and margarine. Turmeric is also used to give a yellow colour to some prepared mustards, canned chicken broths and other foods (often as a much cheaper replacement for saffron).

Momos (Nepali meat dumplings), a traditional dish in South Asia, are spiced with turmeric.

Medicine: In the Ayurvedic medicine, turmeric is thought to have many medicinal properties and many in India use it as a readily available antiseptic for cuts and burns. Whenever there is a cut or a bruise, the home remedy is to reach for turmeric powder. Ayurvedic doctors say it has fluoride which is essential for teeth. It is also used as an antibacterial agent.

It is taken in some Asian countries as a dietary supplement, which allegedly helps with stomach problems and other ailments. It is popular as a tea in Okinawa, Japan. It is currently being investigated for possible benefits in Alzheimer's disease, cancer and liver disorders.

It is only in recent years that Western scientists have increasingly recognised the medicinal properties of turmeric. According to a 2005 article in the Wall Street Journal titled, "Common Indian Spice Stirs Hope," research activity into curcumin, the active ingredient in turmeric, is exploding. Two hundred and fifty-six curcumin papers were published in the past year according to a search of the U.S. National Library of Medicine. Supplement sales have increased 35% from 2004, and the U.S. National Institutes of Health has four clinical trials underway to study curcumin treatment for pancreatic cancer, multiple myeloma, Alzheimer's, and colorectal cancer.

A 2004 UCLA-Veterans Affairs study involving genetically altered mice suggests that curcumin, the active ingredient in turmeric, might inhibit the accumulation of destructive beta amyloids in the brains of Alzheimer's disease patients and also break up existing plaques. "Curcumin has been used for thousands of years as a safe anti-inflammatory in a variety of ailments as part of Indian traditional medicine," Gregory Cole, Professor of medicine and neurology at the David Geffen School of Medicine at UCLA said.

Another 2004 study conducted at Yale University involved oral administration of curcumin to mice homozygous for the most common allele implicated in cystic fibrosis. Treatment with curcumin restored physiologically-relevant levels of protein function.

Anti-tumoral effects against melanoma cells have been demonstrated.

Curry Pharmaceuticals, based in North Carolina, is studying the use of a curcumin cream for psoriasis treatment. Another company is already selling a cream based on curcumin called "Psoria-Gold," which shows anecdotal promise of treating the disease.

A recent study involving mice has shown that turmeric slows the spread of breast cancer into lungs and other body parts. Turmeric also enhances the effect of taxol in reducing metastasis of breast cancer.

Curcumin is thought to be a powerful antinociceptive (pain-relieving) agent. In the November 2006 issue of *Arthritis & Rheumatism*, a study was published that showed the effectiveness of turmeric in the reduction of joint inflammation, and recommended clinical trials as a possible treatment for the alleviation of arthritis symptoms. It is thought to work as a natural inhibitor of the cox-2 enzyme, and has been shown effective in animal models for neuropathic pain secondary to diabetes, among others.

Cosmetics: Turmeric is currently used in the formulation of some sunscreens. Turmeric paste is used by some Indian women to keep them free of superfluous hair. Turmeric paste is applied to bride and groom before marriage in some places of India, where it is believed turmeric gives glow to skin and keeps some harmful bacteria away from the body.

The Government of Thailand is funding a project to extract and isolate tetrahydrocurcuminoids (THC) from turmeric. THCs are colorless compounds that might have antioxidant and skin lightening properties and might be used to treat skin inflammations, making these compounds useful in cosmetics formulations.

Dye: Turmeric makes a poor fabric dye as it is not very lightfast (the degree to which a dye resists fading due to light exposure).

Chemistry: The active substance of turmeric is the polyphenol **curcumin**, also known as C.I. 75300, or Natural Yellow 3. Systematic chemical name is (1*E*,6*E*)-1,7-bis (4-hydroxy-3-methoxyphenyl)-1,6-heptadiene-3,5-dione. It can exist at least in two tautomeric forms, keto and enol. The keto form is preferred in solid phase and the enol form in solution.

Nutmeg: Nutmeg is the actual seed of the tree, roughly egg-shaped and about 20–30 mm long and 15–18 mm wide, and weighing between 5 and 10 grams dried, while mace is the dried "lacy" reddish covering or arillus of the seed.

Several other commercial products are also produced from the trees, including essential oils, extracted oleoresins, and nutmeg butter. The pericarp (fruit/pod) is used in Grenada to make a jam called Morne Delice.

In Indonesia, the fruit is sliced finely, cooked and crystallised to make a fragrant candy called *manisan pala* ("nutmeg sweets").

The most important species commercially is the Common or Fragrant Nutmeg *Myristica fragrans*, native to the Banda Islands of Indonesia; it is also grown in the Caribbean, especially in Grenada. Other species include Papuan Nutmeg *M. argentea* from New Guinea, and Bombay Nutmeg *M. malabarica* from India; both are used as adulterants of *M. fragrans* products.

Culinary Uses: Nutmeg and mace have similar taste qualities, nutmeg having a slightly sweeter and mace a more delicate flavour.

Mace is often preferred in light-coloured dishes for the bright orange, saffron-like colour it imparts. Nutmeg is nice in cheese sauces and is best grated fresh.

In Indian cuisine, nutmeg is used almost exclusively in sweets. It is known as *jaiphal* in most parts of India. It is also used in small quantities in garam masala. In other European cuisine, nutmeg and mace are used especially in potato dishes and in processed meat products; they are also used in soups, sauces and baked goods.

Japanese varieties of curry powder include nutmeg as an ingredient. Nutmeg is a traditional ingredient in mulled cider, mulled wine, and eggnog.

Essential Oils: The essential oil is obtained by the steam distillation of ground nutmeg and is used heavily in the perfumery and pharmaceutical industries. The oil is colourless or light yellow and smells and tastes of nutmeg. It contains numerous components of interest to the oleochemical industry, and is used as a natural food flavouring in baked goods, syrups (*e.g.* Coca Cola), beverages, sweets etc. It replaces ground nutmeg as it leaves no particles in the food.

The essential oil is also used in the cosmetic and pharmaceutical industries for instance in tooth paste and as major ingredient in some cough syrups. In traditional medicine nutmeg and nutmeg oil were used for illnesses related to the nervous and digestive systems. Myristicin and elemicin are believed to be the chemical constituents responsible for the subtle hallucinogenic properties of nutmeg oil. Other known chemical ingredients of the oil are a-pinene, sabinene, a-terpinene and safrole.

Externally, the oil is used for rheumatic pain and, like clove oil, can be applied as an emergency treatment to dull toothache. Put 1–2 drops on a cotton swab, and apply to the gums around an aching tooth until dental treatment can be obtained. In France, it is given in drop doses in honey for digestive upsets and used for bad breath. Use 3–5 drops on a sugar lump or in a teaspoon of honey for nausea, gastroenteritis, chronic diarrhea, and indigestion.

Alternatively a massage oil can be created by diluting 10 drops in 10 ml almond oil. This can be used for muscular pains associated with rheumatism or overexertion. It can also be combined with thyme or rosemary essential oils. To prepare for childbirth, massaging the abdomen daily in the three weeks before the baby is due with a mixture of 5 drops nutmeg oil and no more than 5 drops sage oil in 25 ml almond oil has been suggested.

Nutmeg Butter: Nutmeg butter is obtained from the nut by expression. It is semi solid and reddish brown in colour and tastes and smells of nutmeg. Approximately 75% (by weight) of nutmeg butter is trimyristin which can be turned into myristic acid, a 14-carbon fatty acid which can be used as replacement for cocoa butter, can be mixed with other fats like cottonseed oil or palm oil, and has applications as an industrial lubricant.

History: There is some evidence that Roman priests may have burned nutmeg as a form of incense, although this is disputed. It is known to have been used as a prized and costly spice in medieval cuisine. Saint Theodore the Studite (ca. 758–ca. 826), was famous for allowing his monks to sprinkle nutmeg on their pease pudding when required to eat it. In Elizabethan times it was believed that nutmeg could ward off the plague, so nutmeg was very popular. Nutmeg was traded by Arabs during the Middle Ages in the profitable Indian Ocean trade.

In the late 15th century, Portugal theoretically took over the Indian Ocean trade, including nutmeg, under the Treaty of Tordesillas with Spain and a separate treaty with the sultan of Ternate. But their control of this trade was always only partial and they remained largely participants, rather than overlords. The authority Ternate held over the nutmeg-growing centre of the Banda Islands was quite limited, and the Portuguese failed to gain a serious foothold in the islands themselves.

The trade in nutmeg later became dominated by the Dutch in the 17th century. The British and Dutch engaged in prolonged struggles and intrigue to gain control of Run island, then the only source of nutmegs. At the end of the Second Anglo-Dutch War the Dutch gained control of Run in exchange for the British controlling New Amsterdam (New York) in North America.

The Dutch managed to establish control over the Banda Islands after an extended military campaign that culminated in the massacre or expulsion of most of the islands' inhabitants in 1621. Thereafter, the Banda Islands were run as a series of plantation estates, with the Dutch mounting annual expeditions in local war-vessels to extirpate nutmeg trees planted elsewhere.

As a result of the Dutch interregnum during the Napoleonic Wars, the English took temporary control of the Banda Islands from the Dutch and transplanted nutmeg trees to their own colonial holdings elsewhere, notably Zanzibar and Grenada. Today, a stylised split-open nutmeg fruit is found on the modern national flag of Grenada.

Connecticut gets its nickname ("the Nutmeg State", "Nutmegger") from the legend that some unscrupulous Connecticut traders would whittle "nutmeg" out of wood, creating a "wooden nutmeg" (a term which came to mean any fraud).

World Production: World production of nutmeg is estimated to average between 10,000 and 12,000 tonnes per year with annual world demand estimated at 9,000 tonnes; production of mace is estimated at 1,500 to 2,000 tonnes. Indonesia and Grenada dominate production and exports of both products with a world market share of 75% and 20% respectively. Other producers include India, Malaysia, Papua New Guinea, Sri Lanka and Caribbean islands such as St. Vincent. The principal import markets are the European Community, the United States, Japan and India. Singapore and the Netherlands are major re-exporters.

At one time, nutmeg was one of the most valuable spices. It has been said that in England, several hundred years ago, a few nutmeg nuts could be sold for enough money to enable financial independence for life. The first harvest of nutmeg trees takes place 7–9 years after planting and the trees reach their full potential after 20 years.

Risks and Toxicity: In low doses, nutmeg produces no noticeable physiological or neurological response. Large doses of 30 g or more are dangerous, potentially inducing convulsions, palpitations, nausea, eventual dehydration, and generalized body pain. In amounts of 5–20 g it is a mild to medium hallucinogen, producing visual distortions and a mild euphoria. It is a common misconception that nutmeg contains monoamine oxidase inhibitors (MAOIs).

This is untrue; nutmeg should not be taken in combination with MAOIs but it does not contain them. A test was carried out on the substance which showed that, when ingested in large amounts, nutmeg takes on a similar chemical make-up to MDMA (ecstasy). However, use of nutmeg as a recreational drug is unpopular due to its unpleasant taste and its side effects, including dizziness, flushes, dry mouth, accelerated heartbeat, temporary constipation, difficulty in urination, nausea, and panic. A user will not experience a peak until approximately six hours after ingestion, and effects can linger for up to three days afterwards.

A risk in any large-quantity (over 25 g) ingestion of nutmeg is the onset of 'nutmeg poisoning', an acute psychiatric disorder marked by thought disorder, a sense of impending death, and agitation. Some cases have resulted in hospitalization.

Nutmeg in Literature

Nutmeg appeared to fascinate the 16th-century Europeans, as reflected in this nursery rhyme:

I had a little nut tree,
Nothing would it bear
But a silver nutmeg,
And a golden pear;
The King of Spain's daughter
Came to visit me,
And all for the sake
Of my little nut tree.
Her dress was made of crimson,
Jet black was her hair,
She asked me for my nut tree
And my golden pear.

I said, "So fair a princess
Never did I see,
I'll give you all the fruit
From my little nut tree.

This nursery rhyme is believed to refer to the 1506 visit of the Royal House of Spain to King Henry VII's English court. The 'King of Spain's daughter' refers to the daughter of King Ferdinand and Queen Isabella of Spain. The princess is probably Katherine of Aragon who was betrothed to Prince Arthur, the heir to the English throne. He died, thus Katherine married King Henry VIII.

Prince Arthur was reputed to have deformed genitals (his little nut tree would bear nothing) and the 'silver nutmeg' refers to Britain's spice trade with the East, while the 'golden pear' refers to trade with the West (the golden pear is the ancient Greek Symbol for the Hesperides or West). The Spanish were hoping to gain these by marriage of the Spanish Princess to the British prince, though they were aware there would be no children from the marriage. The last verse is therefore ironic.

Another version has a different ending:

I had a little nut tree,
Nothing would it bear
But a silver nutmeg
And a golden pear.
The King of Spain's daughter
Came to visit me,
And all for the sake
Of my little nut tree.
I skipped over ocean,
I danced over sea,
And all the birds in the air
Couldn't catch me.

The last verse in this version is supposed to refer to Prince Arthur's death before he could marry the Spanish princess.

Clove

Cloves (*Syzygium aromaticum*, syn. *Eugenia aromaticum* or *Eugenia caryophyllata*) are the aromatic dried flower buds of a tree in the family Myrtaceae. It is native to Indonesia and used as a spice in cuisine all over the world. The name derives from French *clou*, a nail, as the buds vaguely resemble small irregular nails in shape. Cloves are harvested primarily in Zanzibar, Indonesia and Madagascar; it is also grown in India, and Sri Lanka.

The clove tree is an evergreen which grows to a height ranging from 10-20 m, having large oval leaves and crimson flowers in numerous groups of terminal clusters. The flower buds are at first of a pale colour and gradually become green, after which they develop into a bright red, when they are ready for collecting. Cloves are harvested when 1.5-2 cm long, and consist of a long calyx, terminating in four spreading sepals, and four unopened petals which form a small ball in the centre.

Uses

Cloves can be used in cooking either whole or in a ground form, but as they are extremely strong, they are used sparingly. The spice is used throughout Europe and Asia and is smoked in a type of cigarettes locally known as *kretek* in Indonesia and in occasional coffee bars in the West, mixed with marijuana to create marijuana spliffs (joints). Cloves are also an important incense material in Chinese and Japanese culture. Clove essential oil is used in aromatherapy and oil of cloves is widely used to treat toothache in dental emergencies.

Cloves have historically been used in Indian cuisine (both North Indian and South Indian). In the north Indian cuisine, it is used in almost every sauce or side dish made, mostly ground up along with other spices. They are also a key ingredient in tea along with green cardamoms. In the south Indian cuisine, it finds extensive use in the biryani dish (similar to the pilaf, but with the addition of local spice taste), and is normally added whole to enhance the presentation and flavour of the rice.

Along with the recreational uses of cloves, they are also said to be a natural anthelmintic.

History

Until modern times, cloves grew only on a few islands in the Maluku Islands (historically called the Spice Islands), including Bacan, Makian, Moti, Ternate, and Tidore. Nevertheless, they found their way west to the Middle East and Europe well before the time of Christ. Archeologists found cloves within a ceramic vessel in Syria along with evidence dating the find to within a few years of 1721 BC.

Cloves, along with nutmeg and pepper, were highly prized in Roman times, and Pliny the Elder once famously complained that "there is no year in which India does not drain the Roman Empire of fifty million sesterces". Cloves were traded by Arabs during the Middle Ages in the profitable Indian Ocean trade. In the late fifteenth century, Portugal took over the Indian Ocean trade, including cloves, due to the Treaty of Tordesillas with Spain and a separate treaty with the sultan of Ternate. The Portuguese brought large quantities of cloves to Europe, mainly from the Maluku Islands. Clove was then one of the most valuable spices, a kg costing around 7 g of gold.

The trade later became dominated by the Dutch in the seventeenth century. With great difficulty the French succeeded in introducing the clove tree into Mauritius in the year 1770; subsequently their cultivation was introduced into Guiana, Brazil, most of the West Indies, and Zanzibar, where the majority of cloves are grown today.

In Britain in the seventeenth and eighteenth centuries, cloves were worth at least their weight in gold, due to the high price of importing them.

The clove has become a commercial 'success', with products including clove drops being released and enjoyed by die-hard clove fans.

Active Compounds

The compound responsible for the cloves' aroma is eugenol. It is the main component in the essential oil extracted from cloves, comprising 72-90%. Eugenol has pronounced antiseptic and anaesthetic properties.

Cinnamon

Cinnamon (*Cinnamomum verum*, synonym *C. zeylanicum*) is a small evergreen tree 10-15 meters (32.8-49.2 feet) tall, belonging to the family Lauraceae, native to Sri Lanka and Southern India. The bark is widely used as a spice. The leaves are ovate-oblong in shape, 7-18 cm (2.75-7.1 inches) long. The flowers, which are arranged in panicles, have a greenish colour, and have a rather disagreeable odour. The fruit is a purple one-centimetre berry containing a single seed.

Its flavour is due to an aromatic essential oil which makes up 0.5 to 1% of its composition. This oil is prepared by roughly pounding the bark, macerating it in sea-water, and then quickly distilling the whole. It is of a golden-yellow colour, with the characteristic odour of cinnamon and a very hot aromatic taste. The pungent taste and scent come from cinnamic aldehyde or cinnamaldehyde and, by the absorption of oxygen as it ages, it darkens in colour and develops resinous compounds. Chemical components of the essential oil include ethyl cinnamate, eugenol, cinnamaldehyde, beta-caryophyllene, linalool and methyl chavicol.

The name cinnamon comes from Greek *kinnámômon*, from Phoenician and akin to Hebrew *qinnâmôn*, itself ultimately from a Malaysian language, cf. Malay and Indonesian *kayu manis* "sweet wood".

History

Cinnamon has been known from remote antiquity, and it was so highly prized among ancient nations that it was regarded as a gift fit for monarchs and other great potentates. It was imported to Egypt from China as early as 2000 BC, and is mentioned in the Bible in Exodus 30:23, where Moses is commanded to use both sweet cinnamon and cassia, and in Proverbs 7:17-18, where the lover's bed is perfumed with myrrh, aloe and cinnamon. It is also alluded to by Herodotus and other classical writers. It was commonly used on funeral pyres in Rome, and the Emperor Nero is said to have burned a year's supply of cinnamon at the funeral for his wife Poppaea Sabina, in 65 AD.

In the Middle Ages, the source of cinnamon was a mystery to the Western world. Arab traders brought the spice via overland trade routes to Alexandria in Egypt, where it was bought by Venetian traders from Italy who held a monopoly on the spice trade in Europe. The disruption of this trade by the rise of other Mediterranean powers such as the Mameluk Dynasties and the Ottoman Empire was one of many factors that led Europeans to search more widely for other routes to Asia.

Portuguese traders finally discovered Ceylon (Sri Lanka) at the end of the fifteenth century, and restructured the traditional production of cinnamon by the *salagama* caste. The Portuguese established a fort on the island in 1518, and protected their own monopoly for over a hundred years.

Dutch traders finally dislodged the Portuguese by allying with the inland Ceylon kingdom of Kandy. They established a trading post in 1638, took control of the factories by 1640, and expelled all remaining Portuguese by 1658. "The shores of the island are full of it", a Dutch captain reported, "and it is the best in all the Orient: when one is downwind of the island, one can still smell cinnamon eight leagues out to sea" (Braudel 1984, p. 215).

The Dutch East India Company continued to overhaul the methods of harvesting in the wild, and eventually began to cultivate its own trees.

The British took control of the island from the Dutch in 1796. However, the importance of the monopoly of Ceylon was already declining, as cultivation of the cinnamon tree spread to other areas, the more common cassia bark became more acceptable to consumers, and coffee, tea, sugar and chocolate began to outstrip the popularity of traditional spices.

Cultivation

Cinnamon is harvested by growing the tree for two years and then coppicing it. The next year a dozen or so shoots will form from the roots. These shoots are then stripped of their bark which is left to dry. Only the thin (0.5 mm) inner bark is used; the outer woody portion is removed, leaving metre long cinnamon strips that curl into rolls ("quills") on drying; each dried quill comprises strips from numerous shoots packed together. These quills are then cut to 5-10 cm long pieces for sale.

Cinnamon comes from Sri Lanka, and the tree is also grown commercially at Tellicherry in southern India, Java, Sumatra, the West Indies, Brazil, Vietnam, Madagascar, Zanzibar, and Egypt. Sri Lanka cinnamon is a very thin smooth bark, with a light-yellowish brown colour, a highly fragrant odour.

Cinnamon and Cassia

The name *cinnamon* is correctly used to refer to Ceylon Cinnamon, also known as "true cinnamon" (from the botanical name *C. verum*). However, the related species Cassia (*Cinnamomum aromaticum*) and Cinnamomum burmannii are sometimes sold labelled as cinnamon, sometimes distinguished from true cinnamon as "Indonesian cinnamon" or, at least for Cassia, "Bastard cinnamon". Ceylon cinnamon, using only the thin inner bark, has a finer, less dense and more crumbly texture, and is considered to be less strong than cassia. Cassia is generally a medium to light reddish brown, is hard and woody in texture, and is thicker (2-3 mm thick), as all of the layers of bark are used. Most of the cinnamon sold in supermarkets in the United States is actually cassia. European health agencies have recently warned against consuming high amounts of cassia, due to a toxic component called coumarin. This is contained in much lower dosages in Ceylon cinnamon and in Cinnamomum burmannii. Coumarin is known to cause liver and kidney damage in high concentrations.

The two barks when whole are easily distinguished, and their microscopic characteristics are also quite distinct. Cinnamon sticks (or quills) have many thin layers and can easily be made into powder using a coffee or spice grinder whereas cassia sticks are much harder, made up of one thick layer, capable of damaging a spice or coffee grinder. It is a bit harder to tell powdered cinnamon from powdered cassia. When powdered bark is treated with tincture of iodine (a test for starch), little effect is visible in the case of pure cinnamon of good quality, but when cassia is present a deep-blue tint is produced, the intensity of the coloration depending on the proportion of cassia.

Cinnamon is also sometimes confused with Malabathrum (*Cinnamomum tamala*) and Saigon Cinnamon (*Cinnamomum loureiroi*).

Uses

Cinnamon bark is widely used as a spice. It is principally employed in cookery as a condiment and flavouring material, being largely used in the preparation of some kinds of desserts, chocolate, spicy candies, tea, hot cocoa and liqueurs. In the Middle East, it is often used in savoury dishes of chicken and lamb. In the United States, cinnamon and sugar are often used to flavour cereals, bread-based dishes, and fruits, especially apples; a cinnamon-sugar mixture is even sold separately for such purposes. Cinnamon can also be used in pickling. Cinnamon bark is one of the few spices which can be consumed directly.

In medicine it acts like other volatile oils and once had a reputation as a cure for colds. It has also been used to treat diarrhea and other problems of the digestive system. Cinnamon is high in antioxidant activity (PMID 16190627, PMID 10077878). The essential oil of cinnamon also has antimicrobial properties (PMID 16104824). This property may allow cinnamon to extend the shelf life of foods.

In the media, "cinnamon" has been reported to have remarkable pharmacological effects in the treatment of type II diabetes. However, the plant material used in the study (PMID 14633804) was actually cassia, as opposed to true cinnamon. Please refer to cassia's medicinal uses for more information about its health benefits. Cinnamon has traditionally been used to treat toothache and fight bad breath and its regular use is believed to stave off common cold and aid digestion.

Cinnamon is used in the system of Thelemic Magick for the invocation of Apollo, according to the correspondences listed in Aleister Crowley's work *Liber 777*.

Cinnamon is also used as an insect repellent. It is widely used when a manufactured insecticide is not wanted or cannot be used because of possible health side effects or allergies.

Allspice

Allspice, also called Jamaica pepper, Myrtle pepper, pimento, or newspice, is a spice which is the dried unripe fruit of the *Pimenta dioica* plant. The name "allspice" was coined by the English, who thought it combined the flavour of several spices, such as salt, chili powder, and garlic.

Flavour

Allspice has a complex aroma, hence its name. It is an aromatic spice with a taste similar to a combination of cinnamon, cloves and nutmeg, but hotter and more peppery.

History

Christopher Columbus discovered allspice in the Caribbean. Although he was seeking pepper, he had never actually seen real pepper and he thought allspice was it. He brought it back to Spain, where it got the name "pimienta," which is Spanish for pepper. Its Anglicized name, pimento, is occasionally used in the spice trade today. Before World War II, allspice was more widely used than it is nowadays. During the war, many trees producing allspice were cut, and production never fully recovered. Most allspice is produced in Jamaica, but some other sources for allspice include Guatemala, Honduras, as well as Mexico. Jamaican allspice is considered to be superior due to its higher oil content, which gives it a more appealing flavour.

Preparation/Form

Allspice is not, as is mistakenly believed by some people who have only come across it in ground form, a mixture of spices. Rather, it is the dried fruit of the *Pimenta dioica* plant. The fruit is picked when it is green and unripe, traditionally they are then sun dried. When dry they are brown and look like large brown peppercorns.

Allspice is most commonly sold as whole dried fruits or as a powder. The whole fruits have a longer shelf-life than the powdered product and produce a more aromatic product when freshly ground before use. Fresh leaves are also used where available: they are similar in texture to bay leaves and are thus infused during cooking and then removed before serving. Unlike bay leaves, they lose much flavour when dried and stored. The leaves and wood are often used for smoking meats where allspice is a local crop.

Uses

Allspice is one of the most important ingredients of Caribbean cuisine. It is used in Caribbean jerk seasoning (the wood is used to smoke jerk in Jamaica, although the spice is a good substitute), in mole sauces, and in pickling; it is also an ingredient in commercial sausage preparations and curry powders. Allspice is also indispensable in Middle Eastern cuisine, particularly in the Levant where it is used to flavour a variety of stews and meat dishes. In Palestinian cuisine, for example, many main dishes call for allspice as the sole spice added for flavoring. Allspice is commonly used in Great Britain and appears in many dishes, including in cakes. Even in many countries where allspice is not very popular in the household, such as Germany, it is used in large amounts by commercial sausage makers. Allspice is also a main flavour used in barbeque sauces.

Allspice has also been used as a deodorant, 18th century Russian soldiers would put allspice in their boots.

Folklore suggests that allspice provides relief for digestive problems.

Volatile oils found in the plant contain eugenol, a weak antimicrobial agent (Yaniv, Sohara et al. 2005).

Cultivation

Allspice is a small shrubby tree, quite similar to the bay laurel in size and form. It can be grown outdoors in the tropics and subtropics with normal garden soil and watering. Smaller plants can be killed by frost, although larger plants are more tolerant. It adapts well to container culture and can be kept as a houseplant or in a greenhouse. The plant is dioecious, hence male and female plants must be kept in proximity in order to allow fruits to develop.

To protect the pimento trade the plant was guarded against export from Jamaica. It is reported that many attempts were made at growing the pimento from seeds, all failed. At one time it was thought that the plant would grow nowhere else except in Jamaica where the plant was readily spread by birds. Experiments were then performed using the constituents of bird droppings, however these were also totally unsuccessful. Eventually it was realized that an elevated temperature, such as that found inside a bird's body, was essential for germinating the seeds.

Camphor

Camphor is a white transparent waxy crystalline solid with a strong penetrating pungent aromatic odour. It is a terpenoid with the chemical formula $C_{10}H_{16}O$. It is found in wood of the **camphor laurel** (*Cinnamonum camphora*), a large evergreen tree found in Asia (particularly in Borneo and Taiwan, hence its alternate name) and some other related trees in the laurel family, notably *Ocotea usambarensis*; it can also be synthetically produced from oil of turpentine. It is used for its scent, as an ingredient in cooking (mainly in India), as an embalming fluid, in religious ceremonies and for medicinal purposes. A major source of camphor in Asia is Camphor basil.

History

The word camphor derives from the French word *camphre*, itself from Medieval Latin *camfora*, from Arabic *kafur*, from Malay *kapur Barus* meaning "Barus chalk". In fact Malay traders from whom Indian and Middle East merchants would buy camphor called it *kapur*, "chalk" because of its white colour. Barus was the port on the western coast of the Indonesian island of Sumatra where foreign traders would call to buy camphor. In the Indian language Sanskrit, the word 'karpoor' is used to denote Camphore. A south-indian adaptation of this word, 'karpooram' has been used for camphor in many south-indian/dravidian languages (like Telugu, Tamil, Kannada and Malayalam)

Camphor was first synthesized by Gustaf Komppa in 1903. Previously, some organic compounds (such as urea) had been synthesized in the laboratory as a proof of concept, but camphor was a scarce natural product with a worldwide demand. The synthesis was the first industrial total synthesis, when Komppa began industrial production in Tainionkoski, Finland, in 1907.

Norcamphor is a camphor derivative with the three methyl groups replaced by hydrogen.

Other substances deriving from trees are sometimes wrongly sold as camphor.

Camphor Trees are widely found in very deep jungles of Western Ghats of Tamil Nadu and Kerala states in South India.

Uses

Modern uses include as a plasticizer for cellulose nitrate, as a moth repellent, as an antimicrobial substance, in embalming, and in fireworks. Camphor crystals are also used to prevent damage to insect collections by other small insects. A form of anti-itch gel currently on the market uses camphor as its active ingredient. It is also used in medicine. Camphor is readily absorbed through the skin and produces a feeling of cooling similar to that of menthol and acts as slight local anesthetic and antimicrobial substance. Camphor is an active ingredient (along with menthol) in vapour-steam products, such as Vicks VapoRub, and it is effective as a cough suppressant. It may also be administered orally in small quantities (50 mg) for minor heart symptoms and fatigue.

In the 17th Century, it was used by Auenbrugger in the treatment of mania.

To prevent camphor from evaporating, just add few Black Peppers into the container of Camphor.

Cockroachs, Snakes and other poisonous insects won't come near the camphor as camphor's strong smell drives them away and the camphor is poisonous for insects.

Camphor is also used in the Mahashiva ratri celebrations of Shiva, the Hindu god of destruction of evil. It's natural pitch substance burns cool without leaving an ash residue, which symbolizes the consciousness.

Culinary

Currently, Camphor is mostly used as a flavoring for sweets in Asia. In ancient and medieval Europe it was widely used as ingredient for sweets but it is now mainly used for medicinal purposes. It is thought that camphor was used as a flavouring in confections resembling ice cream in China during the Tang dynasty (A.D. 618-907). Camphor is widely used in cooking (mainly for desert dishes) in India where it is known as *Pachha Karpooram* (literally meaning "Raw camphor" though "Pachha" means "Green" in Tamil). It is widely available at Indian grocery stores and is labelled as "Edible Camphor." In Hindu poojas and ceremonies, camphor is burned in a ceremonial spoon for performing aarti. This type of camphor is also sold at Indian grocery stores but it is not suitable for cooking. The only type that should be used for food are those which are labelled as "Edible Camphor."

Toxicology

In larger quantities, it is poisonous when ingested and can cause seizures, confusion, irritability, and neuromuscular hyperactivity. In 1980, the United States Food and Drug Administration set a limit of 11% allowable camphor in consumer products and totally banned products labelled as camphorated oil, camphor oil, camphor liniment, and camphorated liniment (but "white camphor essential oil" contains no significant amount of camphor). Since alternative treatments exist, medicinal use of camphor is discouraged by the FDA, except for skin-related uses, such as medicated powders, which contain only small amounts of camphor.

Nigella Sativa

Nigella sativa is an annual flowering plant, native to southwest Asia. It grows to 20-30 cm tall, with finely divided, linear (but not thread-like) leaves. The flowers are delicate, and usually coloured pale blue and white, with 5-10 petals. The fruit is a large and inflated capsule composed of 3-7 united follicles, each containing numerous seeds. The seed is used as a spice.

Nigella sativa seed is known variously as kalonji, kezah (Hebrew), charnushka (Russian), otu (Turkish), habbah Albarakah, (literally *seeds of blessing* Arabic) or siyah daneh (Persian). In English it is called fennel flower, black caraway, nutmeg flower, Roman coriander, or black onion seed. Other names used, sometimes misleadingly, are onion seed and black sesame (both of which are similar-looking but unrelated). Frequently the seeds are referred to as black cumin, this is, however, also used for a different spice, Bunium persicum. It is also sometimes just referred to as nigella or black seed. An old English name *gith* is now used for the corncockle.

This potpourri of vernacular names for this plant reflects that its widespread use as a spice is relatively new in the English speaking world, and largely associated with immigrants from areas where it is well known. Increasing use is likely to result in one of the names winning out, hopefully one which is unambiguous.

Nigella sativa has a pungent bitter taste and a faint smell of strawberries. It is used primarily in candies and liquors. The variety of naan bread called Peshawari naan is as a rule topped with kalonji seeds. In herbal medicine, *Nigella sativa* has hypertensive, carminative, and anthelminthic properties.

Historical Account

According to Zohary and Hopf, archeological evidence about the earliest cultivation of *N. sativa* "is still scanty", but they report seeds of this condiment have been found in several sites from ancient Egypt including Tutenkhamen's tomb. Although its exact role in Egyptian culture is unknown, we do know that items entombed with a pharaoh were carefully selected to assist him in the after life.

The earliest written reference to *N. sativa* is found in the book of Isaiah in the Old Testament. Isaiah contrasts the reaping of nigella with wheat (Isaiah 28: 25, 27). Easton's bible dictionary clarifies that the Hebrew word for nigella, ketsah, refers to without doubt *N. sativa*. According to Zohary and

Hopf, *N. sativa* "was another traditional condiment of the Old World during classical times; and its black seeds were extensively used to flavour food."

In the Unani Tibb system of medicine, *N. sativa* has been regarded as a valuable remedy in a number of diseases. Ibn Sina, most famous for his volumes called *The Canon of Medicine* regarded by many as the most famous book in the history of medicine, refers to nigella as the seed that stimulates the body's energy and helps recovery from fatigue and dispiritedness and several therapeutic effects on digestive disorders, gynecological diseases and respiratory system have been ascribed to the seeds of N. sativa (Ave-sina). It is also included in the list of natural drugs of 'Tibb e nabwi', or prophetic medicine, according to the tradition "hold onto the use of the black seeds for in it is healing for all diseases except death" (Sahih Bukhari vol. 7 book 71 # 592).

The seeds have been traditionally used in the Middle East and Southeast Asian countries to treat ailments including Asthma, Bronchitis, Rheumatism and related inflammatory diseases, to increase milk production in nursing mothers, to promote digestion and to fight parasitic infections. Its oil has been used to treat skin conditions such as eczema and boils and to treat cold symptoms. The many uses of nigella has earned for this ancient herb the Arabic approbation 'Habbatul barakah' meaning the seed of blessing.

Use in Folk Medicine

Nigella sativa has been used for centuries, both as a herb and pressed into oil, by people in Asia, Middle East, and Africa for medicinal purposes. It has been traditionally used for a variety of conditions and treatments related to respiratory health, stomach and intestinal health, kidney and liver function, circulatory and immune system support, and for general overall well-being.

In Islam, it is regarded as one of the greatest forms of healing medicine available. The prophet Muhammad once stated that the black seed can heal every disease— except death.

2

Characteristics of Steroid Yielding Plants

Introduction: India has a rich heritage of plant based drugs both for use in preventive and curative medicines. Steroids and their related active metabolites are of great value in drug and pharmaceutical industry. They have numerous and diversified physiological functions and pharmacological effects such as influence on carbohydrate, protein, fat and purine metabolism; on electrolyte and water balance; on the functional capacities of the cardiovascular system viz., kidney, skeletal, muscle, nervous system and some organs and tissues.

The term steroid (= sterol like) is derived from sterol (In Greek, Stereos= solid and ol=alcohol) as most of these compounds contain alcoholic group. All the steroids are structurally related and mostly saturated, colourless compounds found in plants and animals. Steroid includes a variety of compounds, among which sapogenins hold a very important position. Sapogenins when linked with sugar constitutes the saponins. Saponins are natural products, which have the property of forming soapy leather when shaken with water.

Production of steroid drugs is a large scale industry (Applezweig, 1962). In 1967, total world consumption of steroids precursors was one thousand tones, two third of which came from diosgenin and the remaining one third from the variety of miscellaneous sources. Other steroidal alkaloids that could become available in large quantities are tomatidine, Solasodine and Neotigogenin. Till today, more than four thousand plant species have been investigated which has resulted in the identification of some thirty naturally occurring steroids sapogenins many of which could provide valuable source materials for steroids compounds.

Steroidal Sapogenin Yielding Plants

A. Diosgenin Source

S. N.	*Name of Plant*	*Part used*
1	Allium fuscoviolacenum	Bulbs
2	Allium narcissifolium	Bulbs
3	Aspidistra elatior	Under ground parts
4	Balanites roxburghii	Fruits and leaves
5	Convallaria keisukei	Under ground parts
6	Costus speciosus	Rhizome
7	Dioscorea composita	Rhizome
8	Dioscorea floribunda	Rhizome
9	Dioscorea deltoidea	Rhizome
10	Dioscorea gracillima	Rhizome
11	Dioscorea polystachya	Rhizome
12	Dioscorea prazeri	Rhizome
13	Dioscorea sativa	Rhizome
14	Dioscorea septembola	Rhizome
15	Funkia ovata	Leaves
16	Kallstroemia pubescens	Whole plant
17	Ophiopogon japonicus	Tuber
18	Paris polyphyalla	Tuber
19	Polygonatum latifolium	Leaves
20	Polygonatum multiflorum	Leaves
21	Smilax exfelsa	Leaves
22	Solanum introsum	Fruits
23	Solanum indicum	Fruits
24	Tamas communis	Under ground parts
25	Tribulus terrestris	Over ground parts
26	Trigonella foenum	Leaves and seeds
27	Trigonella tschonoskii	Under ground parts

B. Solasodine Source

S.N.	Name of Plant	Part Used
1	Solanum eleagnifolium	Fruit
2	Solanum jubatum	Fruit
3	Solanum incanum	Fruit
4	Solanum khasianum	Fruit
5	Solanum laciniatum	Fruit, Leaves and stem
6	Solanum mammosum	Fruit
7	Solanum marginatum	Fruit and Leave
8	Solanum platanifolium	All parts
9	Solanum sodomaeum	Fruit, leaves and bud
10	Solanum tomentosum	Leaves
11	Solanum trachysyphyum	Fruit and Leaves
12	Solanum trilobatum	Fruit
13	Solanum verbascifolium	Fruit
14	Solanum xanthocarpum	Fruit

C. Hecogenin Sources

S.N.	Name of Plant	Part Used
1	Agave species	Leaves

D. Yamogenin Sources

S.N.	Name of Plant	Part Used
1	Asparagus officinalis	Roots
2	Smilax aspera	Leaves
3	Trigonella foenum graceum	Roots and Leaves

Commercially source material for steroids is only few species belonging mainly to the genus Dioscorea and Solanum. Although diosgenin has been identified in other species such as Costus speciosus, Trigonella foenum graceum and Kallstromia pubescens but there is no evidence at present that they would be interesting commercially, and therefore, they have not been described in detail. Efforts have been directed towards the cultivation of several Solanum species as the source material for the production of steroids. Genus Dioscorea, with over 600 species is widely distributed in tropical world, except few species in temperate.

Some of the species like Dioscorea alata and Dioscorea esculenta have been cultivated for a long for their edible tubers. There are about 15 species of this genus, which are known to contain steroidal sapogenins chiefly diosgenin. In the world, Mexico, Guatemala, Costa Rico, India and China are the major diosgenin producing countries.

Most of the world production of diosgenin today is met from Central American species mainly Dioscorea floribunda and D. Composita. The total turnover of bulk steroids in the world is estimated to be about 500 million US dollars and estimated world usage to be somewhere between 550-650 tones of diosgenin. In India, Dioscorea deltoidea and D. Prazeri occurring in North-West and North-East Himalayas respectively are the natural sources of diosgenin.

Species Characteristics of Steroid Yielding Plants

Dioscorea Deltoidea Wall

It occurs throughout the North Western Himalayas extending from Kashmir and Punjab eastwards to Nepal and China at the altitude of 900-3000 meters above msl. It completes growth cycle in five years. It is an extensive climber with unarmed stem twining to the left. Leaves alternate, rhizome horizontal, scattered roots, skin light brown. Part used is rhizome and harvesting is done after three years during December, at dormant stage. Diosgenin varies from 2-5% on dry weight basis.

Dioscorea Prazeri Prain and Burkill

The plant occurs in wet parts of Eastern Himalayas including North Bihar, West Bengal, Nepal, Sikkim, Bhutan and Abhore hills upto 5500 meters and prefer well drained soils particularly river banks. It is a climber with smooth or slightly ridged, unarmed stem twining to the left. Leaves are alternate or rarely opposite. Part used is rhizome which is short rather stout, gray brown to nearly black, creeping horizontally. Diosgenin varies between 2-5% on dry weight basis.

Dioscorea Floribunda Mart and Gal

It was introduced in India from Central America and is now grown in parts of Karnataka, Assam and Goa. Like D. Deltoidea, it is also perennial vine and life cycle goes for 1-4 years. Part used is rhizome and diosgenin content lies between 3-3.5% on dry weight basis. Two years crop is found more economical and therefore two years old plant yield 2.5-3.0 kg rhizome.

Dioscorea Composita Hemsl

It also is a native to Central America and is grown successfully under Jammu conditions in India. The plant is quite hardy and vigorous which completes its life cycle in 1-5 years. The highest gains in tuber growth are obtained only after 4-5 years. Average diosgenin content is 2-4% on dry weight basis. Among Dioscorea deltoidea, D. Floribunda and D. Composita, the later is preferred for commercial production of diosgenin. Moreover, diosgenin obtained from its tuber has highest purity.

Uses: Diosgenin after converted into 16-Dehydro-pregnenolon acetate is most widely used as an active ingredient in preparation of many steroid drugs, sex hormones and oral contraceptive pills. Saponins of Dioscorea are used for washing silk, wool and hair, and as fish poison. They are also reported to kill lice. Cortisone prepared from these species is used in rheumatic diseases and ophthalmic disorders.

Dioscorea spp., which are commercial source of diosgenin, has limitations in ensuring large supplies on a sustained basis due to its restricted distribution in few localities. It becomes necessary to search for an alternative botanical source, which could be easily cultivated under a wide range of agroclimatic conditions and provide the industry with the raw material at comparative price. Costus speciosus satisfies all the criteria of such a substitute.

Costus Speciosus (Koenig) Sm

It is a common plant with a tuberous rhizome, distributed throughout India up to an elevation of 4000 meters amsl. It is 4-10 meters in height with large lanceolate leaves about one foot in length. Flowers are in red colour with white limbs and yellowish centres. It is often cultivated as ornamental plant. Part used is rhizome which constitutes average diosgenin 2-4% on dry weight basis.

Uses: The rhizome is edible and is used for cooking purpose and is mucilaginous without aroma. It is rich in starch but the fibre content is high when compared with other tuber food. The rhizome is used for tonic purpose and as anthelmintic in Uttar Pradesh.

Trigonella Foenum Graceum Linn

An aromatic annual, about 30-60 cm tall is found wild in Kashmir, Punjab and upper gangetic plains and also cultivated in many parts of India. Seeds are the source of two steroidal sapogenins namely diosgenin and gitogenin. The presence of few more sapogenins including yamogenin has also been reported.

The seeds are used as condiment and for flavouring the food preparations. Diosgenin was first raw material source to be used for high volume production (Djerassi, 1966) because it was available in a readily purified form and at sufficiently high volume that was cheaply collected.

Solasodine, as a nitrogen analogue of diosgenin, seems to be in a strong competitive position with diosgenin itself. Indeed, solasodine derived from Solanum laciniatum is reported to be the sole source of cortisone and progesterone in the USSR (Alekseenko et al., 1976). In India, Solanum khasianum and certain other species are being cultivated for the local production of solasodine for the use in Indian pharmaceutical industry. Solasodine occurs mainly in the genus Solanum. This genus comprises about 2000 species distributed in the warmer regions of the world. About 22 species are endemic to India.

Solanum Khasianum Clarke

It is widely distributed in the Indian sub-continent extending from sea level to 2000 meters and is reported from Khasi, Jaintia and Naga hills of Assam and Manipur and in Arunachal Pradesh up to 1850 meters. It also occurs in Sikkim, West

Bengal, Orrisa, Upper Gangetic plains, lcwer hills of Himalayas and in Nilgiris to an altitude of 1600 meters. It is reported from North-East, North-West, Southern as well as Central India and extends up to Burma and China.

It is a stout, much branched under shrub varying in height between 0.75m to 1.5m with almost straight prickles, leaves ovate and lobed. Lobes triangular and prickly on both the surfaces. The flowers are white. The berries are yellowish or greenish. The seeds are smooth brown and compressed. Part used is berry and solasodine content lies between 1-3% on dry weight basis. The main limitation of this species is that it bears spines that are quite vicious. Moreover solasodine is obtained only from berries. Therefore this species is paving way for the use of Solanum laciniatum and Solanum aviculare in the commercial utilization.

Soalnum Laciniatum Ait

Commonly known as Kangaroo apple and was introduced in India from Russia. It is a perennial shrub but mostly grows up to two years. It is about 2 meters in height with long trifurcated dark green leaves and purplish stem and branches. The flowers are purplish blue. Berries are borne in bunches of 5-7 with dark green colour but turn to yellowish orange colour at maturity. Seeds are small flat, round and brownish in colour. Part used are leaves, stem and berries. Leaves contain solasodine content to 1-3.8% and berries (unripe greenish yellow) contain 3.5-4.0% of solasodine on dry weight basis. Solanum khasianum and S. Laciniatum are worth considering for foliar production of solasodine.

Uses: Solasodine is used in production of sex hormones and oral contraceptive pills.

Agave Linn

Agave is a large genus with short stemmed half woody plant species, bearing a rosette of long, erect, pointed and fleashy leaves. In various species like A. Americana, A. Cantala, A. Sisalana, A. Angustifolia, leaves yield a valuable fibre.

Uses: Hecogenin is used for making sex hormones and oral contraceptive pills.

From the foregoing facts, it is clear that in order to establish and support a broad based steroid industry, it is imperative to start large scale cultivation of various species like Dioscorea composita and D. floribunda and development of high yielding varieties and mutants *i.e.* Solanum khasianum to ensure sustainable supply of source material.

Medicinal, Aromatic and Cosmetic (MAC) Plants

Medicinal Plants in Health

Various trees, shrubs, herbs, climbers and creepers/climbers, grass, succulents, bulbs and rhizomes are mainly used to prepare traditional medicines. The specific parts of the plant that make the medicines include bark, roots (tuber), leaves and buds. The preparation of herbal medicine varies for 'external' and' internal' illnesses.

A large number of perceived diseases have been reported to be mainly treated through the application of specific traditional herbal medicine. These include: head, tooth and gum aches, sore eyes, growths on the face, common colds, and dandruffs, brain fatigue, tonsillitis, mumps, mouth sores and aching ears. Also, neck stiffness, asthma, coughs, chest pains, pneumonia, tuberculosis, and whooping cough belong to this category of diseases.

Stomach ailments treated by herbal medicine include acidity, ulcers, worms, heartburn, diarrhoea, constipation, amoeba, poisons, anthrax, nausea and cholera. Backaches, joint aches, swollen legs, sprains and rheumatism are also among the diseases treated by traditional plant-based medicines. Special herbal remedies are reported for malaria and other kinds of fevers, rashes, boils, measles, itching, scurvy, skin growths, dry skin and ringworms. Similarly, venereal diseases, fresh cuts, wounds from poisoned arrows, burns, anaemia, diabetes and high blood pressure are mostly treated by traditional herbal medicines.

Antenatal herbal treatment include birth control; abortifecients and menstrual overflow while post-natal treatments include problems related to afterbirths and excessive bleeding.

Medicinal Plants in Culture

Plants in Meru have been part of the local people's culture for as long as they have known them. There are particular trees that are believed to give long life - the Mugumo tree; those that give healing by just singing praises to them (Mutuntu) and those that bring prosperity and health to couples and families (Kirao).

Cultural diversity is also manifest in Meru people views on herbal medicines. The differential perceptions are influenced by a variety of factors. These include socio-demographic *e.g.* ethnicity, religion; psyco-social *e.g.* knowledge, attitudes and beliefs; and enabling factors *e.g.* socio-economic status and profession of respondents.

Cosmetic and Aromatic Plants in Health and Culture

Although fewer people tend to use plant-based products nowadays due to the already available cosmetic and aromatic products found at modern chemists, there is recently a reorientation towards the use of cosmetic plants. Some parts of Kenya still use wild plants for their cosmetic products, but the Meru people only knows these specific plants from the past. The main reported uses then include traditional perfumes for circumcised girls and women. Among young children, particular roots of cosmetic plants are crushed and the powder mixed with saliva and applied on the body of a child, also to cure colds and coughs. An example of such a plant is the Ndago plant.

Medicinal and Aromatic Plants

Which well known plant never touches the ground, does not follow a 12-month vegetation cycle, stays green year round, blooms in the winter, and sells predominately in December? The answer, of course, is mistletoe. Current research questions the efficacy of this highly controversial plant. "Rejected by clinical oncologists but used by practitioners and cancer patients, it is applied as a remedy to treat a broad spectrum of different diseases, such as epilepsy, diabetes, hypertension, arthrosis, hepatitis, HIV infection, labour pains, and cancer."

Now a new book on the therapeutic uses and industrial applications of Viscum has been published. Rarely mentioned in traditional books on herbal medicine mistletoe research remains questionable. Because the "extracts may exert different effects than purified substances" individual immune responses vary greatly. There is a great need for further investigation. Currently no clinical data are available documenting long-term therapy treatment.

Whether the extracts of Viscum become a major player in the fight against cancer, this book makes for provocative reading. Researchers in pharmacognosy and phystochemistry will find this book documented with references to hundreds of research articles invaluable. While most articles feature the European point of view, there is one article from Japan and another from South Africa. Although none of the articles originate from the United States, American research is well represented in the bibliographies, as are traditional Chinese uses for this herb.

Responding to the increased demand for information on medicinal and aromatic plants this fascinating look at this highly controversial plant is the 16th volume in the series Medicinal and Aromatic Plants Industrial Profiles. This series brings together articles scattered through a variety of sources, is international in scope, and includes many little known sources. Each article is well documented and is introduced by the editor Arndt Bussing, head of the Department of Applied Immunology at the foundation Krebsforschung Herdecke, University of Witten/Herdecke. Mistletoe: the Genus Viscum is illustrated with colour photographs of the plant, line drawings, and chemical structures. With few exceptions most references are current, dating from 1990 to 2000.

While this book would be of interest to scientists in botany, agriculture, and phytochemistry, those working in alternative medicine, pharmaceutical, and health sciences should find it of greater interest. Recommended for academic and research libraries.

Aromaticity

Aromaticity is a chemical property in which a conjugated ring of unsaturated bonds, lone pairs, or empty orbitals exhibit a stabilization stronger than would be expected by the stabilization of conjugation alone. It can also be considered a manifestation of cyclic delocalization and of resonance .

This is usually considered to be because electrons are free to cycle around circular arrangements of atoms, which are alternately single- and double-bonded to one another. These bonds may be seen as a hybrid of a single bond and a double bond, each bond in the ring identical to every other. This commonly-seen model of aromatic rings, namely the idea that benzene was formed from a six-membered carbon ring with alternating single and double bonds (cyclohexatriene), was developed by Kekule. The model for benzene consists of two resonance forms, which corresponds to the double and single bonds' switching positions. Benzene is a more stable molecule than would be expected without accounting for charge delocalization.

Theory: By convention, the double-headed arrow indicates that the two structures are simply hypothetical, since neither is an accurate representation of the actual compound. The actual molecule is best represented by a hybrid (average) of these structures, which can be seen at right. A C=C bond is shorter than a C—C bond, but benzene is perfectly hexagonal—all six carbon-carbon bonds have the same length, intermediate between that of a single and that of a double bond.

A better representation is that of the circular o bond (Armstrong's inner cycle), in which the electron density is evenly distributed through a o bond above and below the ring. This model more correctly represents the location of electron density within the aromatic ring.

The single bonds are formed with electrons in line between the carbon nuclei—these are called sigma bonds. Double bonds consist of a sigma bond and another bond—a o bond. The o-bonds are formed from overlap of atomic p-orbitals above and below the plane of the ring. The following diagram shows the positions of these p-orbitals:

Since they are out of the plane of the atoms, these orbitals can interact with each other freely, and become delocalised. This means that instead of being tied to one atom of carbon, each electron is shared by all six in the ring. Thus, there are not enough electrons to form double bonds on all the carbon atoms, but the "extra" electrons strengthen all of the bonds on the ring equally. The resulting molecular orbital has o symmetry.

History: The first known use of the word "aromatic" as a chemical term—namely, to apply to compounds that contain the phenyl radical—occurs in an article by August Wilhelm Hofmann in 1855. If this is indeed the earliest introduction of the term, it is curious that Hofmann says nothing about why he introduced an adjective indicating olfactory character to apply to a group of chemical substances, only some of which have notable aromas. Ironically, many of the most odoriferous organic substances known are terpenes, which are not aromatic in the chemical sense. But terpenes and benzenoid substances do have a chemical characteristic in common, namely higher unsaturation indexes than many aliphatic compounds, and Hofmann may not have been making a distinction between the two categories.

The cyclohexatriene structure for benzene was first proposed by August Kekule in 1865. Over the next few decades, most chemists readily accepted this structure, since it accounted for most of the known isomeric relationships of aromatic chemistry. However, it was always puzzling that this purportedly highly unsaturated molecule was so unreactive toward addition reactions.

An explanation for this exceptional stability is conventionally attributed to Sir Robert Robinson, who was apparently the first (in 1925) to coin the term aromatic sextet as a group of six electrons that resists disruption.

In fact, this concept can be traced further back, via Ernest Crocker in 1922, to Henry Edward Armstrong, who in 1890, in an article entitled The structure of cycloid hydrocarbons, wrote the (six) centric affinities act within a cycle...benzene may be represented by a double ring (sic)... and when an additive compound is formed, the inner cycle of affinity suffers disruption, the contiguous carbon-atoms to which nothing has been attached of necessity acquire the ethylenic condition.

Here, Armstrong is describing at least four modern concepts. Firstly, his "affinity" is better known nowadays as the electron, which was only to be discovered seven years later by J.J. Thomson. Secondly, he is describing electrophilic aromatic substitution, proceeding (thirdly) through a Wheland intermediate, in which (fourthly) the conjugation of the ring is broken. He introduced the symbol C centred on the ring as a shorthand for the inner cycle, thus anticipating Eric Clar's notation. Arguably, he also anticipated the nature of wave mechanics, since he recognized that his affinities had direction, not merely being point particles, and collectively having a distribution that could be altered by introducing substituents onto the benzene ring (much as the distribution of the electric charge in a body is altered by bringing it near to another body). The quantum mechanical origins of this stability, or aromaticity, were first modelled by Hückel in 1931.

Characteristics of aromatic (Aryl) compounds: An aromatic compound contains a set of covalently-bound atoms with specific characteristics:

1. A delocalized conjugated o system, most commonly an arrangement of alternating single and double bonds
2. Coplanar structure, with all the contributing atoms in the same plane
3. Contributing atoms arranged in one or more rings
4. A number of o delocalized electrons that is even, but not a multiple of 4. This is known as Hückel's rule. Permissible numbers of o electrons include 2, 6, 10, 14, and so on
5. Special reactivity in organic reactions such as electrophilic aromatic substitution and nucleophilic aromatic substitution

Whereas benzene is aromatic (6 electrons, from 3 double bonds), cyclobutadiene is not, since the number of o delocalized electron is 4, which of course is a multiple of 4. The cyclobutadienide (2–) ion, however, is aromatic (6 electrons). An atom in an aromatic system can have other electrons that are not part of the system, and are therefore ignored for the 4n + 2 rule. In furan, the oxygen atom is sp^2 hybridized. One lone pair is in the o system and the other in the plane of the ring (analogous to C-H bond on the other positions). There are 6 o electrons, so furan is aromatic.

Aromatic molecules typically display enhanced chemical stability, compared to similar non-aromatic molecules. The circulating o electrons in an aromatic molecule produce ring currents that oppose the applied magnetic field in NMR. The NMR signal of protons in the plane of an aromatic ring are shifted substantially further down-field than those on non-aromatic sp2 carbons. This is an important way of detecting aromaticity. By the same mechanism, the signals of protons located near the ring axis are shifted up-field. Planar monocyclic molecules containing 4n o electrons are called antiaromatic and are, in general, destabilized. Molecules that could be antiaromatic will tend to alter their electronic or conformational structure to avoid this situation, thereby becoming non-aromatic. For example, cyclo-octatetraene (COT) distorts itself out of planarity, breaking o overlap between adjacent double bonds. Mobius aromaticity describes a special case of aromaticity.

Aromatic molecules are able to interact with each other in so-called o -o stacking: the o systems form two parallel rings overlap in a "face-to-face" orientation. Aromatic molecules are also able to interact with each other in an "edge-to-face" orientation: the slight positive charge of the substituents on the ring atoms of one molecule are attracted to the slight negative charge of the aromatic system on another molecule.

Many of the earliest-known examples of aromatic compounds, such as benzene and toluene, have distinctive pleasant smells. This property led to the term "aromatic" for this class of compounds, and hence to "aromaticity" being the eventually-discovered electronic property of them.

Aromatic Compound Classifications: The key aromatic hydrocarbons of commercial interest are benzene, toluene, ortho-xylene and para-xylene. About 35 million tonnes are produced worldwide every year. They are extracted from complex mixtures obtained by the refining of oil or by distillation of coal tar, and are used to produce a range of important chemicals and polymers, including styrene, phenol, aniline, polyester and nylon.

Heterocyclics: In heterocyclic aromatics, one or more of the atoms in the aromatic ring is of an element other than carbon. This can lessen the ring's aromaticity, and thus (as in the case of furan) increase its reactivity. Other examples include pyridine, imidazole, pyrazole, oxazole, thiophene, and their benzannulated analogs (benzimidazole, for example).

Polycyclics: Polycyclic aromatic hydrocarbons (PAH) are molecules containing two or more simple aromatic rings fused together by sharing two neighbouring carbon atoms (see also simple aromatic rings). Examples are naphthalene, anthracene and phenanthrene.

Substituted Aromatics: Many chemical compounds contain simple aromatic rings in their structure. Examples are DNA which contains purine and pyrimidine, trinitrotoluene (TNT), acetylsalicylic acid (aspirin) and paracetamol.

Aromaticity in Other Systems: Aromaticity is found in ions as well: the cyclopropenyl cation (2e system), the cyclopentadienyl anion (6e system), the tropylium ion (6e) and the cyclooctatetraene dianion (10e). Aromatic properties have been attributed to non-benzenoid compounds such as tropone. Aromatic properties are tested to the limit in a class of compounds called cyclophanes.

A special case of aromaticity is found in homoaromaticity where conjugation is interrupted by a single sp3 hybridized carbon atom. When carbon in benzene is replaced by other elements in borabenzene, silabenzene, germanabenzene, stannabenzene, phosphorine or pyrylium salts the aromaticity is still retained. Aromaticity is also not limited to compounds of carbon, oxygen and nitrogen.

Metal aromaticity is believed to exist in certain metal clusters of aluminium. Mobius aromaticity occurs when a cyclic system of molecular orbitals formed from p-o atomic orbitals and populated in a closed shell by 4n (n is an integer) electrons is given a single half-twist to correspond to a Mobius topology. Because the twist can be left-handed or right-handed, the resulting Mobius aromatics are dissymmetric or chiral. Up to now there is no doubtless proof, that a Mobius aromatic molecule was synthesized. Aromatics with two half-twists corresponding to the paradromic topologies first suggested by Johann Listing have been proposed by Rzepa in 2005. In carbo-benzene the ring bonds are extended with alkyne and allene groups.

Aromatic Hydrocarbon

An aromatic hydrocarbon (abbreviated as AH) or arene is a hydrocarbon, the molecular structure of which incorporates one or more planar sets of six carbon atoms that are connected by delocalised electrons numbering the same as if they consisted of alternating single and double covalent bonds. The term 'aromatic' was assigned before the physical mechanism determining aromaticity was discovered, and was derived from the fact that many of the compounds have a sweet scent. This sweet scent actually came from impurities in the compounds (which are not actually aromatic in the sense initially described). The configuration of six carbon atoms in aromatic compounds is known as a benzene ring, after the simplest possible aromatic hydrocarbon, benzene. Aromatic hydrocarbons can be monocyclic or polycyclic.

Note: Some non-benzene-based compounds which follow Hückel's rule are also aromatic compounds. Examples of non-benzene compounds with aromatic properties are furan, a heterocyclic compound with a five-membered ring which includes an oxygen atom, and pyridine, a heterocyclic compound with a six-membered ring containing one nitrogen atom.

Benzene Ring Model: Benzene, C_6H_6, is the simplest AH and was recognized as the first aromatic hydrocarbon, with the nature of its bonding first being recognized by Friedrich August Kekule von Stradonitz in the 19th century. Each carbon atom in the hexagonal cycle has four electrons to share. One goes to the hydrogen atom, and one each to the two neighbouring carbons. This leaves one to share with one of its two neighbouring carbon atoms, which is why the benzene molecule is drawn with alternating single and double bonds around the hexagon.

Many chemists draw a circle around the inside of the ring to show that there are six electrons floating around in delocalized molecular orbitals the size of the ring itself. This also accurately represents the equivalent nature of the six bonds all of bond order ~1.5. This equivalency is well explained by resonance forms. The electrons float above and below the ring, and the electromagnetic fields they generate keep the ring flat. General properties:

1. Display aromaticity.
2. The Carbon-Hydrogen ratio is very large.
3. They burn with a sooty yellow flame because of the high carbon-hydrogen ratio.
4. They undergo electrophilic substitution reactions and nucleophilic aromatic substitutions.

Arene synthesis: Many laboratory methods exist for the organic synthesis of arenes from non-arene precursors:

- Alkyne trimerization, [2+2+2] cyclization of three alkynes
- Dotz reaction
- Diels-Alder reactions of alkynes with pyrone or cyclopentadienone with expulsion of carbon dioxide or carbon monoxide.
- Aromatization of cyclohexanes and other aliphatic rings: reagents are, catalysts used in hydrogenation such as platinum, palladium and nickel (reverse hydrogenation), quinones and the elements sulfur and selenium.
- Bergman cyclization, enyne plus hydrogen donor

Arene reactions: The main arene reactions are:

- Electrophilic aromatic substitution
- Nucleophilic aromatic substitution
- Many coupling reactions to biraryls
- Hydrogenation to saturated rings

Lesser known reactions:

- Unusual thermal Diels-Alder reactivity of arenes can be found in the Wagner-Jauregg reaction
- Other photochemical cycloaddition reactions with alkenes through excimers.

Benzene and derivatives of benzene: Benzene derivatives have from one to six substituents attached to the central benzene core. Examples of benzene compounds with just one substituent are phenol which carries a hydroxyl group and toluene with a methyl group. When there is more than one substituent present on the ring their spatial relationship becomes important for which the arene substitution patterns ortho, meta and para are devised. For example three isomers exist for cresol because the methyl group and the hydroxyl group can be placed next to each other (ortho), one position removed from each other (meta) or two positions removed from each other (para). Xylenol has two methyl groups in addition to the hydroxyl group and for this structure 6 isomers exist.

Examples of benzene derivative with alkyl substituents (alkylbenzenes) are:

- Ethylbenzene C_6H_5-CH_2-CH_3
- Mesitylene $C_6H_3(-CH_3)_3$
- Toluene C_6H_5-CH_3
- Xylene $C_6H_4(-CH_3)_2$

Examples of other aromatic compounds:

- Aniline C_6H_5-NH_2
- Acetylsalicylic acid $C_6H_4(-O-C(=O)-CH_3)(-COOH)$
- Benzoic acid C_6H_5-COOH
- Biphenyl $(C_6H_5)_2$
- Chlorobenzene C_6H_5-Cl
- Nitrobenzene C_6H_5-NO_2
- Paracetamol $C_6H_4(-NH-C(=O)-CH_3)(-OH)$
- Phenacetin $C_6H_4(-NH-C(=O)-CH_3)(-O-CH_2-CH_3)$
- Phenol C_6H_5-OH
- Picric acid $C_6H_2(-OH)(-NO_2)_3$
- Salicylic acid $C_6H_4(-OH)(-COOH)$
- Trinitrotoluene $C_6H_2(-CH_3)(-NO_2)_3$

The arene ring has an ability to stabilize charges. This is seen in, for example, phenol (C6H5-OH), which is acidic at the hydroxyl (OH), since a charge on this oxygen (alkoxide -O-) is partially delocalized into the benzene ring.

Polycyclic aromatic hydrocarbons: Some important arenes are the polycyclic aromatic hydrocarbons (PAH); they are also called polynuclear aromatic hydrocarbons. They are composed of more than one aromatic ring. The simplest PAH is benzocyclobutene (C_8H_6).

Common examples are Naphthalene, Anthracene, Phenanthrene and triphenylene. More exotic examples are helicenes and Corannulene.

Simple Aromatic Ring

Simple aromatic rings are aromatic organic compounds (also known as arenes or aromatics) that consist only of conjugated planar ring systems with delocalized pi electron clouds instead of discrete alternating single and double bonds. Typical simple aromatic compounds are benzene and indole.

Simple aromatic rings can be heterocyclic if they contain non-carbon ring atoms, *e.g.* oxygen, nitrogen, or sulfur. Simple monocyclic aromatic rings are usually five-membered rings like pyrrole or six-membered rings like pyridine. Fused aromatic rings like naphthalene or purine consist of monocyclic rings that share their connecting bonds.

The nitrogen (N) containing aromatic rings can be separated into non-basic and basic aromatic rings:

- In the non-basic rings the lone pair of electrons of the nitrogen atom is delocalized and contributes to the aromatic pi electron system. In these compounds the nitrogen atom is connected to a hydrogen atom. Examples of non-basic nitrogen-containing aromatic rings are pyrrole and indole.
- In the basic aromatic rings the lone pair of electrons is not part of the aromatic system and extends in the plane of the ring. This lone pair is responsible for the basicity of these nitrogenous bases, similar to the nitrogen atom in amines. In these compounds the nitrogen atom is not connected to a hydrogen atom. Examples of basic aromatic rings are pyridine or quinoline. Several rings contain basic as well as non-basic nitrogen atoms, *e.g.* imidazole and purine. Under acidic conditions these compounds get protonated and form aromatic cations (*e.g.* pyridinium).

In the oxygen (O) and sulfur (S) containing aromatic rings one of the electron pairs of the heteroatoms contributes to the aromatic system (similar to the non-basic nitrogen containing rings), while the second lone pair extends in the plane of the ring (similar to the basic nitrogen containing rings).

Criteria for Aromaticity:

- Molecule must be cyclic.
- Every atom in the ring must have a "p" orbital which overlaps with "p" orbitals on either side (completely conjugated).
- Molecule must be planar.
- It must contain an odd number of pairs of pi electrons; must satisfy Huckel's rule: (4n+2) pi electrons, where n is an integer starting at zero.

In contrast, molecules with 4n pi electrons are antiaromatic.

3

Culinary Herbs and Aromatic Plants

Consumption Pattern

Americans are consuming ever increasing amounts of fresh, frozen, processed and dried culinary herbs and spices, and this trend appears to be here to stay. The same trend is true for specially fruits and vegetables (Fielding 1988). Factors accounting for increased consumption include interest in new foods and tastes, availability of more fresh herbs, advertising and promotion to food services and institutional food chains, and expanding ethnic populations demanding foods and flavourings of their homeland.

Who will be supplying these herbs and are there opportunities for commercial growers in the production of dried and fresh herbs? Much of the dried herbs produced domestically are produced in California by well-established food companies that own and operate drying and processing facilities and already package, transport and market these products. Growth in this area will continue as long as increased demand and consumption of these herbs continue. Additional growth is likely to occur in the contract growing of herbs by private growers to supply raw product to drying and processing companies.

Some companies both grow and process their own product, but most contract practically all of their raw material needs to growers. Processing companies that are now procuring most of their dried herbs abroad may be more willing to obtain some of the same materials domestically Growth in the dried herbal market will also probably occur with an increasing number of spice companies and natural food wholesalers and retailers catering to specialized markets (*e.g.* organic or pesticide free-herbs and spices, specially restaurants) and which unlike many of the larger food and flavor houses produce specialized herb and other food products.

There has been tremendous growth in the fresh herb market as evidenced by the increased variety of herbs available both in the larger supermarkets, the smaller grocery outlets, farmers markets, and roadside farm markets (Simon 1986, Simon et al. 1989, Simon and Clavio 1989, Simon and Grant 1987a, b). Herbs that were only available dried, or fresh during a few months of the year, are now being marketed fresh cut and more recently, as live potted herbs in the produce sections of supermarkets all year long. Recognizing this growth, the USDA (1989c) now lists weekly prices for herbs sold in nineteen major wholesale markets plus the type of container, package, and weight count, and quality of each unit in the National Market News Report. The herbs now covered include anise, arrugala, basil, borage, chervil, chives, cilantro, dill ginger root horseradish, parsley lemongrass, marjoram, mint, oregano, rosemary savoury, sage, sorrel tarragon, thyme, and watercress.

The successful introduction of new culinary herbs into commercial production requires a purposeful strategy and a solid information base. Unfortunately culinary herbs and essential oil crops have been studied little compared to all other food and fiber crops (Craker et al. 1986). While several extension guides have been published on herbs, few guides based on research are available in this country In a bibliographic review of the scientific literature from 1971-1980 (Simon et al. 1984), over 10,000 authors are listed with published research articles on the major economical herbs of the temperate zone involving horticultural research (38%), botany (17%), chemistry (14%), pharmacology (11%), ecology and germplasm (8%). With the exception of peppermint and spearmint most all crop research on herbs was conducted outside of the United States. Although the United States is the principal world producer of mint oils, only 10% of all published mint research from 1971-1980 originated in the U.S. (Craker et al. 1986).

Promising Herbs

There is a wide range of culinary herbs that can be grown in the continental United States and which may offer potential for production. Many herbs are already being commercially produced, albeit in small quantities, often in relatively small farms. Those herbs which show promise for the fresh market are listed. Three examples of culinary herbs with great promise are discussed below.

Coriander (Coriandrum sativum L): This annual herb native to the eastern Mediterranean and southern European region has long been prized for its spicy aromatic seeds which are used either whole or in ground form as a main ingredient in curry and other food and flavor products. Coriander can be grown as a seed crop in the U.S. using existing mechanization and production technology but seeds ripen unevenly and the mature seeds shatter from the plant. Present demand for coriander seed is met by existing foreign suppliers and although the yield of coriander seed is moderately high (1,100-1,700 kg/ha) and the cost of production relatively low, there is still a question whether domestic commercial opportunities exist for coriander seed production as a spice. The profit margin of coriander would at best match the more traditional cash crops (maize, soybeans). Postharvest costs of cleaning the seed, handling and shipping can be major factors determining the profitability of this seed spice crop. Coriander seed is also processed via steam distillation for the extractable essential oil of which d-linalool is the major constituent. The oil is then used in the food and perfume industries.

Recently, American consumers have witnessed the introduction of coriander leaves into the marketplace. This fresh product, known as cilantro, is marketed in bunches as a leafy green spice. While new to American cuisine, cilantro has long been a popular herb in Oriental, Middle Eastern and Latin American cooking.

Coriander, a cool season crop, is easy to grow as a culinary herb and is most suited to fertile loam soils. The plant is direct seeded with a seed drill at rates of 13-18 kg/ha in very early spring. In Florida and New Jersey, coriander is often planted weekly At harvest, the whole plant is manually cut and bunched in the field.

One of the major problems in producing cilantro is premature flowering. Bolting becomes acute as the days get hotter and longer. A number of seed companies now offer slow-to-bolt (long-standing) cultivars. There are significant differences among coriander cultivars regarding the response to premature flowering, and while some are less susceptible, none are totally unresponsive to high temperatures and long days (Simon et al. 1989). Thus, cilantro is planted as a spring, early summer, or fall crop.

The aroma of cilantro is also due to an extractable essential oil, although its composition is distinctly different from the seed oil. Quality of fresh cilantro is based upon strong green colour, strong aroma, and visual appearance (*i.e.* freedom from insects, discolorations). To the grower, yield and the cultivars' resistance to bolt are additional factors to be considered. Cilantro has a relatively short shelf life and requires refrigeration. Cilantro can be kept for 3 to 4 weeks at 0°C, but only 2 to 3 weeks when stored at 5°C (Cantwell 1989). Cilantro is routinely iced after harvest. Cilantro is expected to become increasingly important in the U.S. due in part to the expanding Hispanic and Arabic populations, its unique flavor, and increasing familiarity in the marketplace.

Sweet Fennel (Foeniculum vulgare Mill.): Sweet fennel has highly aromatic leaves and attractive green fern-like foliage but is best known for its seeds which are sold commercially as a spice. Limited domestic production for seed has occurred periodically, but demand is relatively small and adequate supplies can be obtained abroad. Successful domestic production of fennel for the seed as a spice will probably not occur unless the yields can be significantly improved, supplies from abroad become limited, or a government programme makes the production of new crops more beneficial.

Fennel is a perennial but grown as an annual. It is most suited to well drained light loam soil. The plant is easy to grow and is typically direct seeded (3.5-5 kg/ha seed/acre) into the ground in beds with a specialized planter adapted to small-seeded crops. Plant spacing varies significantly with rows in the beds 60-1 00 cm apart and with final plant stands of 10-3 cm apart in the row. Fennel is a cool-season crop, seeds are sown in early spring and germinate at temperatures >7°C (optimum soil temp. approx. 16-18°C). Yields of up to 2,240 kg/ha have been achieved, although earlier USDA estimates were only in the range of 650-900 kg/ha (Sievers 1948). The plant requires 100-115 days to mature before harvest.

The production of fennel as a culinary herb, cultivated both for its aromatic leaves and enlarged leaf stalk is on the rise. This type, called Florence fennel or finocchio fennel, is a different subspecies than regular fennel produced as a seed spice. Very popular in Europe as a specially vegetable in many culinary dishes, it is commonly consumed raw in Italy and cooked in France. Finocchio is becoming commonplace in U.S. supermarkets and consumer interest and familiarity is increasing. One of the limiting factors to increased consumption is the public's unfamiliarity with it's preparation, use and taste. Unfortunately finocchio fennel is often marketed under the misnomer of anise, another culinary herb (Pimpinella anisum L.), which has led to market and consumer confusion. Both plants contain high amounts of anethole in the essential oil, imparting the licorice-like aroma and taste.

The time to harvest fennel bulbs is difficult to assess because the thickened leaf stalk continues to grow and develop until flowering takes place. Care in harvesting, grading and packing fennel must be taken to ensure a high quality fresh pack. Harvesting, cleaning, trimming and packing is done by hand. The foliage must be dark green and fresh in appearance and the stalk and bulb (enlarged base of leaf stalk) a lighter greenish-white colour. The bulb must be firm and the product free from insects and discolorations. Once harvested, fennel should be kept at 0 to 2°C (Seelig 1974). The plants are retailed individually, either wrapped in plastic or simply displayed like celery.

Great variability (in growth and aroma) in commercially available cultivars of fennel and finocchio fennel exist (Simon et al. 1989) making the proper selection of cultivars for spring and fall production important. Finocchio fennel shows excellent potential for future growth in the U.S.

Oregano (Origanum spp.): Their has been a significant increase in the consumption of oregano for both the fresh and processed market (Tucker 1987). Oregano, the common name for a wide number of plant species with a characteristic aroma and flavor, is a perennial aromatic plant native to the dry calcareous soils of southern Europe, southwest Asia, and the eastern Mediterranean (Simon et al. 1984). A major problem which has limited domestic production was in the difficulty in distinguishing the many plant species and types of oregano imported and marketed as oregano. Imported oregano was found to be derived from 16 plant genera and more than 40 plant species (Calpouzos 1954), resulting in oregano being described as a flavor and aroma rather than an individual plant. Taxonomic work by Tucker (1986, 1989) has identified the major types of commercial cultivars and cultivated taxa in this country and the major types of imported oregano. Yet much of the imported oregano arrives as a blend of plants. Selection of an individual line for domestic production, particularly for the dried leaf or as an essential oil, remains difficult.

The European type of oregano comes mainly from subspecies of O. vulgare L. including ssp. hirtum (Link) Ietswaart, ssp. virens (Hoffmanns. & Link) Ietswaart and ssp. viride (Boiss.) Hayek (Tucker 1989). In contrast Mexican oregano, also called Mexican sage, is principally gathered from the small Mexican shrub, Lippia graveolens H.B.K. (Simon et al. 1984), although leaves from other species are collected.

The essential oil of European oregano is composed mainly of carvacrol and thymol. The range of each can be very wide and many chemotypes are available. The herb or the extracted oil is used in a variety of meat and sausage products, salads, stews, sauces and soups. European oregano and to a larger extent Mexican oregano, are used in flavoring Mexican foods, pizza, and barbecue sauces.

Oregano is generally transplanted to the field and grown on light, dry well-drained soils for periods of 3 to 6 years.

Domestic horticultural studies on this species are limited. Although yields of more than 14 tonnes fresh herb/ha or almost 4 tonnes dried herb/ha were obtained from one commercial line by a single annual harvest (Simon et al. 1989), typically yields are much lower (1.5-3 tonnes dried herb/ha). Plants can be harvested multiple times each year (from 2 to 6) depending upon the location and end-use. Opportunities exist for dried product as well as for the fresh market. Once harvested for the fresh market oregano should be kept at 0deg.C to maximize shelf-life (Cantwell 1989).

Prospects

Production of culinary herbs for the fresh, frozen processed and dried market will likely increase. The large growth in the production of fresh culinary herbs provides opportunities to growers that either develop a market niche or cooperate closely with a broker or specialist in marketing. It is likely that the large volume herbs will continue to come from areas of intensive vegetable production such as Florida, New Jersey and California. Herbs can be expected to become fully integrated with fresh market vegetables in packaging, cooling, transport, and marketing operations. Unless governmental regulations change, there will be strong competition from Mexico, the Caribbean, and other areas to supply fresh herbs to the American public. Overproduction of specific herbs within a limited marketplace can result in significant decreases in the wholesale market prices. Greater opportunities for small producers maybe in the development of specialized markets, rather than for the wholesale trade.

Supercritical Fluid Extraction (SFE)

The supercritical fluid extraction (SFE) has been applied only recently to sample preparation on an analytical scale. This technique resembles Soxhlet extraction except that the solvent used is a supercritical fluid, substance above its critical temperature and pressure. This fluid provides a broad range of useful properties. One main advantage of using SFE is the elimination of organic solvents, thus reducing the problems of their storage and disposal in the lipidologist laboratory.

Furthermore, several legislative protocols (such as the EPA Pollution Prevention Act in the USA) have focused on advocating a reduction in the use of organic solvents which could be harmful to the environment.

Besides ecological benefits, one of the most interesting properties of SFE is the high diffusion coefficients of lipids in supercritical fluids, far greater than in conventional liquid solvents. Thus, the extraction rates are enhanced and less degradation of solutes occurs.

Several studies have shown that SFE is a replacement method for traditional gravimetric techniques. In addition, carbon dioxide, which is the most adopted supercritical fluid has low cost, is a nonflammable compound and devoid of oxygen, thus protecting lipid samples against any oxidative degradation.

Principles for the Analytical SFE of Lipids

The first guiding principle is the optimization of the solubility of lipids in supercritical CO_2 and the improvement of the fractionation with respect to a particular lipid species.

Important data on the solubility of vegetal oils and other lipids may be found in the detailed study of Stahl et al. (Dense gases for extraction and refining, Springer Verlag, Heidelberg, 1987). These data have led to perform oil and fat extractions above 600 bar and temperatures from 80 to 100°C.

It should be emphasized that many lipid solutes have similar solubility parameters, making their separation by SFE difficult. An improvement in the separation of complex lipid mixture may be found by the integration of adsorbent compound into the extraction cell with the sample.

Several compounds such as alumina, silica, Celite, Florisil or synthetic resins were proposed for the optimization of lipid differential extraction.

The improvement of lipid SFE needs also the study of the kinetics of the lipid removal from the sample matrix. It must be noticed that the fast back-diffusion of analytes in the supercritical fluid reduces the extraction time since the complete extraction step is performed in about 20 min instead of several hours.

A common practice in SFE, which must be mentioned in connection with the physicochemical properties of supercritical fluids, is the use of modifiers (co-solvents). These are compounds that are added to the primary fluid to enhance extraction efficiency.

Thus, the addition of 1 to 10% of methanol or ethanol to CO2 expands its extraction range to include more polar lipids. When the extraction was performed with supercritical carbon dioxide and 20% of ethanol, more than 80% of the phospholipids were recovered from salmon roe (Tanaka Y et al., J Oleo Sci 2004, 53, 417).

Instrumentation

Those wishing to build their own experimental equipment should read the detailed study of Hawthorne et al. (in Practical supercritical chromatography and extraction, Caude M., Thiebaut D, Eds, Harwood Academic, 1999).

ISCO Inc was one of the first companies to address the off-line SFE market. Extraction cells of 0.5 up to 15 ml are offered.

An automatic version permits automated valve operation for extraction of one or two samples and another model permits 24 samples to be automatically and sequentially extracted. ISCO has also offered a extraction system (FastFat HT) specifically made for the rapid determination of fat content in foods and agriculture products ("The Isco FastFat HT provides rapid, accurate % fat determination in a wide range of foods-a critical parameter in quality control, product labeling, and calibrating on-line process control equipment.

With FastFat HT, you get reliable results in minutes, and eliminate costly delays in production decisions").

Applied Separation offers several extraction units offering great flexibility with respect to sample size and experimental design. Extractor cell sizes can range from several ml to one liter. Off-line and in-line trapping of solutes may be realized.

IECO Corporation is offering a total fat analyzer designed with a triple parallel channel system ("LECO's new TFE2000 Fat/Oil Determinator is specifically designed to determine fat/ oil content and eliminate the need for hazardous chemicals used in Soxhlet, Mojonnier/Roese-Gottlieb, acid hydrolysis, and other solvent extraction methods. Using inexpensive compressed CO2 as the solvent, the analyte is extracted from the sample and transferred to the removable ultra efficient solid phase collection traps. Precise calculations are determined by the integrated balance based on sample weight, and the before and after weights of the collection vials"). Application notes may be found on the LECO site.

The use of high purity SFE-grade CO2 is not required but impurity and moisture in industrial grade CO2 can accumulate and may interfere with further analytical operations (gas or liquid chromatography). Thus, an on-line fluid cleanup system may be used to remove trace contaminants.

Extractions can be performed in static, dynamic or recirculating mode. During static extraction, the cell is filled with the supercritical fluid, pressurized and allowed to equilibrate. In the dynalic mode, the fluid is run continuously through the cell, and in the recirculating mode, the same fluid is repeatedly pumped in the cell before being pumped out to the collection vial.

Important Parameters

A. *Sample Matrix:* The levels of lipid content and moisture are important for the analytical process. Lipid levels may be from 1 up to 50% (w/w).

B. *Sample Preparation:* Moisture may inhibit contact between extraction fluid and sample. Thus, removal of water by freeze drying is recommended prior to SFE.

It may be also efficient to disperse the sample matrix, to grind the sample to increase the mass transfer of lipids. The choice of drying agent can be made by consulting the study of Bulford (Bulford MD et al., J chromatogr A 1993, 657, 413).

C. *Collection of the Lipid Extract:* The collection method for the resultant extract must be optimized to avoid incomplete extraction. The open vials are most frequently used, a sub-ambient cooling being useful for volatile species. It is best to use a collection vial packed with a surface area material, *i.e.* glass beads, glass wool (Snyder J. M. et al., JAOCS 1994, 71, 261) or containing some volume of a chosen solvent. The supercritical CO2 can be separated from the collected analytes without trouble or disposal problems.

Application of SFE to Lipids

Several reviews were devoted to the application of SFE for the extraction of lipids in various sample types. Those of Clifford A et al. (in Supercritical fluid technology in oil and lipid chemistry, AOCS Press, chap. 19, 1996), Eller FJ et al. (Sem Food Technol 1996, 1, 145) and King J.W. (Grasas y Aceites 2002, 53, 8) should be consulted for specific applications.

Food and various agricultural products were successfully analyzed for their fat and levels by SFE. Progressively, SFE may be regarded as an alternative to organic solvent extraction methods. The extraction efficiencies of SFE and organic solvent methods (Soxhlet or liquid-liquid extractions) were frequently compared and shown to be in good agreement (Eller FJ et al., J Agric Food Chem 1998, 46, 3657). It must be noticed that gravimetric-based results can be influenced by the sample matrix, the moisture and non-lipid moieties and the extraction solvent.

Total fat determinations were done in meat products with two different extractors and compared with a standard method (Berg H et al., J AOAC Int 2002, 85, 1064). The amount and the composition agreed well with results from the standard procedure. To obtain quantitative recoveries by SFE, 1 ml ethanol was added to 1 g sample in the extraction cells before extraction.

Extracting conditions largely affected the composition of dissolved lipids in freeze-dried animal samples (Tanaka Y et al., J Oleo Sci 2003, 52, 295). Thus, one group of triglycerides was extracted from salmon roe while another group remained in the matrix together with phospholipids and a large part of astaxanthin. It is now well known that the extraction yield and composition of triglycrides depend on the extracting conditions. This was verified for the extraction of oil from seaweed (Cheung PCK et al., J Agric Food Chem 1998, 46, 4228), tomato seeds (Bhupesh CR et al., J Food Sci Technol 1996, 31, 137) or soyabean oil (Snyder JM et al., JAOCS 1984, 61, 1851).

The extraction and separation of phospholipids from tuna fish have been described using various concentrations of methanol in supercritical CO2 (Tanaka Y et al., J Oleo Sci 2005, 54, 569). Good recovery of DHA-rich phospholipids were claimed in a series of industrial processes.

A detailed description of a reliable procedure adapted for the determination of total fat in milk- and soy-based infant formula powder has been published by LaCroix DE et al. (J AOAC Int 2003, 86, 86).

The extraction of a specific lipid moiety is generally influenced by substances which are co-extracted, all having a high solubility in supercritical CO2.

One technique to overcome this problem is to use a sorbent to retard the analyte of interest, the interfering substances being removed first. Then, a higher CO2 extraction density or a co-solvent is used to removed the analyte of interest from the sorbent. Thus, it was shown that NH2-bonded silica is able to retard sterols.

Analytical SFE has also been used for lipid-derived volatiles such as aroma in various food samples. For the application of SFE to the study of total fat and lipid classes in meats, the studies of Berg H et al. (J Chromatogr A 1997, 785, 345) and Chandrasekar R. (JAOAC int 2001, 84, 466) should be consulted.

Field of the Invention

The extraction of the principal significant components of herb and spice plants containing pigment, flavor, and aroma and, when present in the starting material, antioxidant, using edible, food-grade solvent.

Of especial interest is the extraction of the principal significant components of spices and herbs represented by plants of the family Solanaceae, representatively Capsicums such as paprika, red pepper, and chili, and Lycopersicon, representatively tomato, all containing carotenoid pigments; Umbelliferae, representatively celery, lovage, dill, carrot, cilantro, fennel, cumin, caraway, parsley, angelica, and anise; Compositae, representatively marigold, artemisia, and tarragon; Leguminosae, representatively fenugreek; Labiatae, representatively rosemary, thyme, sage, oregano, marjoram, mint, savoury, and basil; Zingerberacae representatively ginger, cardamom, and turmeric, Lauraceae, representatively laurel, cinnamon, cassia, and bay; Myrtaceae, representatively allspice and clove; of the genus Myristica, representatively mace and nutmeg; of the genus Piper, representatively black and white pepper; of the genus Vanilla, representatively vanilla; of the genus Allium, representatively onion and garlic; of the genus Sesamum, representatively sesame seed; Cruciferae, representatively mustard and horseradish; the defining characteristic being that it is of a spice or herb plant material from which flavor, aroma, colour, and/or antioxidant can be extracted and used to flavor and/or colour foods and beverages or otherwise employed to enhance the palatability of foods and beverages.

Background of the Invention and Prior Art

The present invention relates to a method of increasing the stability and reducing the microbial counts of both spice or herb oleoresin and the residual cake from which the oleoresin has been extracted. The process simultaneously extracts and concentrates the principal flavor, aroma, colour, and other active components, produces a concentrated and standardized food-grade extract of active components, and a standardized food-grade residual solid, with both the extract and residual solids having significantly reduced microbial counts and frequently also improved stability.

Concentrated extracts of spices and herbs are universally used for flavoring and coloring of food, beverages, and pharmaceuticals. These extracts are traditionally used where a standardized, sterile, and uniform concentrate offers the benefits of control which are inherently difficult to obtain from raw spice or herb, or where the bulk of the raw material is not needed or undesirable.

Ground spice and herb solids are universally used for flavoring, coloring, and imparting otherwise favourable characteristics to food and beverages where the bulk, functional characteristics, and appearance of the food or beverage is important.

Dried spices and herbs, most often in their ground form, are used in the preparation of food and beverages to add flavor, aroma, colour, and preservative properties that make the food more palatable and appealing. The dried spices, ground or unground, are usually added to the food or beverage during preparation at such a point in the preparation that time is allowed for the principal components of interest to be extracted into the food or beverage to impart the desired combination of attributes to the food or beverage. Further, as spices and herbs are notoriously known to have inconsistent levels of the flavor, aroma, colour, or antioxidants, it is commonly required that spices of varying levels of the principal components of interest be blended to make a final product that is consistent with regard to the principal components of interest to achieve predictable and repeatable performance with respect to the flavor, aroma, colour, or antioxidant release into the food or beverage system in which they are used. This is a costly and time consuming process.

As suggested in prior art, much of the flavor, aroma, and/or colour often is not effectively transferred to the food or beverage. U.S. Pat. No. 2,507,084 overcomes this obstacle of under-utilization of the principal components of interest by first extracting the principal components of interest and subsequently coating the spent spice from the extraction process with a portion of the extract originally removed, thereby extending the useful amount of flavor and aroma that can be derived from a given quantity of spice. It is also disclosed that this process derives value from the exhausted spice solids, from which the flavor, aroma, colour, or antioxidants have been removed, which would otherwise be a waste product. This is a complicated and costly process for recovery of the maximum value of the spice and its principal components of interest.

Traditional extraction processes for the manufacture of concentrated extracts (concentrated several fold as compared with the raw material) involve not only the use of various non-edible solvent systems, but also a large proportion of solvent in relation to the compounds of interest. Many require the use of petroleum distillates, chlorinated solvents, or highly flammable solvents which must be eliminated almost completely from the finished products to make them safe for consumption. These systems require expensive distillation equipment and special precautions must be taken to ensure worker safety and to limit environmental impact.

The intensive processing required often destroys, modifies, or loses some of the more unstable compounds, delicate aromas, flavours, or pigments. More significantly, the last traces of undesirable non-edible solvents are very difficult to separate from the concentrated extract. The residual solid must necessarily contain the same residual non-edible solvents, which are removed only with difficulty. Such residual solvents limit the potential use of the residual solid for human consumption, and are potential environmental contaminants.

Other concentration techniques rely on high pressure equipment to obtain good solvating properties from gases, *e.g.*, liquid or supercritical CO2 (U.S. Pat. No. 4,490,398). High pressure liquefied or supercritical gas extraction requires expensive equipment and has limited solvating abilities for some compounds requiring the addition of cosolvents, or solvents such as propane and butane, which are also difficult to control and may be environmentally sensitive or undesirable in a finished product.

Following extraction and desolventization, the concentrated extract is often standardized with edible solvents and emulsifiers to provide a concentrate with reproducible levels of the active or principal compounds of interest to the user. In an effort to overcome the shortcomings and risks associated with the above-mentioned processes, extraction has been carried out using edible solvents such as vegetable oils or lard. Typical extraction procedures are disclosed in U.S. Pat. Nos. 3,732,111; 2,571,867; and 2,571,948. These methods require a relatively large volume of solvent in relation to the compounds of interest and result in a dilute extract which is limited in its application and which has few of the advantages of the concentrates which can be produced using volatile solvents.

U.S. Pat. No. 4,681,769 discloses a method for simultaneously extracting and concentrating in a series of high pressure countercurrent mechanical presses using relatively small amounts of vegetable oil as the solvent in an attempt to overcome the problem of dilution inherent in earlier processes. This method suffers from severe limitations in temperature and pressure ranges in an attempt to avoid unacceptable oxidative damage, colour loss, yield losses, and flavor changes with the final result being that contact times must be unduly extended for up to 16-24 hours, adding greatly to the cost of the process. Extraction cycle times are unduly long for a given size pressing operation, and the process does not provide for a controlled degree of browning or for sterilization of the extract or of the residual solid. It is also limited to temperatures of less than 100° F. to avoid alleged undue oxidation and thus it does not allow for the use of edible solvents which have a melting point of more than 100° F. or which are highly viscous at temperatures of less than 100° F. Maximum pressures of up to about 500 PSI (cone pressure) are claimed and this severely limits the efficiency and throughput rate for a given size pressing operation, as shown by the disclosure of this patent.

Traditional methods for the sterilization of ground spices and herbs involve the use of extremely toxic substances such as ethylene oxide or methyl bromide, irradiation, or steam and moisture treatment to reduce plate counts to less than 100,000. Chemical sterilization and irradiation of spices and herbs are disagreeable to the consumer because of the perceived risk of residual chemicals and/or radiation remaining in the plant matter and, as a result, several processes using added moisture, such as water or steam, at elevated pressures have been developed as alternatives. Typical sterilization procedures are disclosed in U.S. Pat. Nos. 4,210,678, 4,790,995, and 4,910,027. All sterilization processes are inherently costly in that they require a separate processing step or steps to accomplish the sterilization, and also present the possibility of further degrading the more unstable components. Addition of moisture or water vapour, as disclosed in U.S. Pat. Nos. 4,210,678 and 4,910,027, prior to or during the heating and sterilization process results in a cooked aroma not typical of the fresh, dehydrated spice or herb and also results in steam distillation and loss of some of the volatile flavor and aroma constituents.

U.S. Pat. Nos. 4,790,995 and 4,910,027 require the addition of a coating of animal protein to protect the spice from the loss of volatile aroma compounds during the sterilization process with water vapour. U.S. Pat. No. 4,210,678 requires bringing the moisture of the spice to above 8-14%, in some cases up to 16-20%, and holding the spice for an extended period of time prior to sterilization to equilibrate the moisture. This additional step is costly and time consuming. In the case of Capsicums, severe browning and off aromas and flavours are developed in the presence of moistures in excess of 10% at elevated temperatures above 180° F.

Traditional methods for controlling the brownness or degree of caramelization of Capsicum solid to enhance its visual appearance involve the use of elevated temperatures and the addition of vegetable or animal fats or oils to bring up the surface colour and luster of the ground spice. This requires a separate and costly processing operation.

Above all, there is the unsolved problem of obtaining satisfactory yields, quality, and throughput rates of acceptable extract having an acceptable content of active principle in the edible solvent without undesirable oxidative damage to, and reduced stability of, the principal compounds of interest, while at the same time providing for simultaneous sterilization of both the herb or spice solid and extract.

Obviously, existing prior art procedures leave much to be desired, and it is a primary objective of the present invention to provide a procedure for the production of sterilized spice and herb products having enhanced stability and which otherwise obviates the shortcomings of the prior art.

Objects of the Invention

Accordingly, it is an object of the present invention to provide a process for simultaneously and rapidly extracting and concentrating the principal components of herb and spice solids, at temperatures of at least 130° F., preferably 130 to about 450° F., in a process which is completely free of petroleum, chlorinated or highly flammable solvent, does not require high pressure gas handling equipment, does not require distillation for solvent removal, uses only food-grade edible solvents which are typically used in the trade to standardize the resulting extract to a desired concentration, and provides a product of reduced bacterial count which is free of adulterants and impurities.

Another object of this invention is to prepare such a concentrated extract by a process which is simple, environmentally friendly, and economical.

A further object of this invention is to prepare a residual solid or press cake which is edible, free of residual petroleum distillates, chlorinated solvent, or other adulterants, which is standardized with respect to the principal components of commercial interest, which has a predictable and controlled degree of brownness or caramelization, and which has a controlled level of water activity with its attendant increased resistance to oxidative deterioration of carotenoid pigments and colour loss where this is otherwise a problem.

Still another object of this invention is to prepare a residual solid or press cake that is standardized with respect to the principal components of interest, that when reground rapidly and efficiently imparts flavor, aroma, colour, and/or other principal components of interest to a food or beverage in which it is used, and all without the use of undesirable non-edible solvents that are inherently difficult to remove from spice solids remaining after extraction prior to standardization with respect to the principal components of interest, are environmentally unfriendly, and are perceived by the consumer as being undesirable in the preparation of a food ingredient. A still further object of this invention is to provide such a process wherein antioxidants can be added to the edible solvent system so as to protect the concentrated extract and the residual solids against oxidative degradation of the principal components of interest, *i.e.,* flavor, aroma, and colour, which are extracted from the raw plant material or left in the residual solids.

Still a further object of this invention is to prepare an edible extract and an edible residual solid with reduced microbial activity by a process wherein the moisture of the herb or spice is kept below 10%, preferably below 8%, thereby avoiding the loss of volatile flavor and aroma constituents and avoiding the development of uncontrolled browning and off flavor development at temperatures in excess of 130° F. which are necessary to effect high extraction efficiencies, reduction in microbial activity, and improved stability of the carotenoid pigments in both the extract and in the residual solids.

Yet a further object of this invention is to prepare an extract with increased resistance to oxidative degradation of pigments and consequent colour loss. Still an additional object is to provide a process wherein and whereby the residual spice or herb plant solids have their tissue ruptured so as to produce quick release of the flavor, aroma, colour, or antioxidant component therein and thereof when in use in a food or beverage thereby greatly enhancing its use effectiveness, and whereby all products of the process may be conveniently standardized with respect to the principal flavor, aroma, colour, or antioxidant component of interest.

Other objects will be apparent to one skilled in the art to which this invention pertains and still others will become apparent hereinafter as the description proceeds.

Brief Description of the Drawings

The process of the present invention, including the several process steps involved in the simultaneous extraction and concentration of herb or spice solids, *e.g.*, Capsicum solids, to produce the desired extract and sterilized residual solid, both of which have increased resistance to oxidative degradation, and which can be readily standardized to desired levels of the principal components of interest. Although the process illustrated comprises three extraction stages, the number of stages can be decreased to two or increased to more than three to effect the desired relative principal component concentration in the extract and in the residual solid.

Summary of the Invention

The invention, then, inter alia, comprises the following, alone or in combination:

A continuous multistage mixing, high pressure pressing, and countercurrent extraction process for the production of a concentrated edible extract and quick-release edible residual solids, both of reduced bacterial content, and both of which contain herb or spice pigment, flavor, and aroma and, when present in the starting material, antioxidant, from herb or spice plant solids, comprising the following steps: subjecting said herb or spice solids to a countercurrent extraction process involving a plurality of mixing and pressing stages, including first and last mixing stages and first and last pressing stages, together with up to about fifty percent by weight of an edible solvent, to produce an extract and residual solids, continuously returning the extract from each pressing stage to the previous mixing stage, and finally separating the extract from the first pressing stage and separating the residual solids from the last pressing stage, all pressing stages being carried out at a temperature of at least 130° F.; such a process wherein the temperature is 130 to about 450° F.; such a process wherein the solids are subjected to internal pressures in the press stages of at least 6,000 pounds per square inch; such a process wherein the weight of the edible solvent is 5% to about 20% by weight of the solids; such a process wherein the moisture content of the starting solids is less than 10% by weight, and wherein bacterial count reduction is effected at this low moisture content, thereby avoiding undesirable loss of volatile flavor and aroma constituents and avoiding the development of cooked, off flavours and aromas which occur at higher moisture contents; such a process wherein the solids extracted in the process are selected from the group consisting of chipotle, turmeric, black pepper, onion, rosemary, and oregano; such a process wherein the edible solvent is selected from the group consisting of soybean oil, corn oil, cottonseed oil, rapeseed oil, peanut oil, mono-, di-, or triglycerides, lecithin, edible essential oils, sesame oil, edible alcohols, hydrogenated or partially hydrogenated fats or oils, polyoxyethylene sorbitan esters, limonene, edible animal fats or oils, mixtures thereof, and edible derivatives thereof; such a process wherein fine particulate solids are filtered or centrifuged from the extract and alternatively discarded, returned to a mixing or pressing stage of the process, or incorporated in the final residual solids; such a process which includes the steps of hydrating the final extract to add water to the extent of 5% to 200% by weight of the gums and fine particulate solids therein and filtering or centrifuging to remove said gums and solids; such a process including the step of returning the separated hydrated gums and solids to the final residual solids; such a process including the step of rehydrating the final residual solids with water to a water activity greater than 0.3 AW for stabilization thereof; such a process wherein the solids are rehydrated to a water activity of about 0.4 to 0.6 AW; such a process wherein an effective stabilizing amount of an edible antioxidant or chelator is included in the edible solvent; such a process wherein the antioxidant comprises an antioxidant selected from the group consisting of lecithin, ascorbic acid, citric acid, tocopherol, ethoxyquin, BHA, BHT, TBHQ, tea catechins, sesame, and the antioxidant activity from an herb of the Labiatae family; such a process wherein the antioxidant comprises a naturally-occurring antioxidant from an herb of the family Labiatae or powdered ascorbic acid; such a process wherein the antioxidant comprises the antioxidant activity from an herb selected from the group consisting of rosemary, thyme, and sage; such a process wherein the temperature is greater than 180° F.; and such a process wherein the temperature is between about 180° F. and 235° F.

Moreover, an extract of herb or spice plant solids produced by the process having a high level of principal flavor, aroma, colour, or antioxidant components of interest and a low bacterial count due to the high temperature employed in its production and due to the low water content not greater than 10% in the starting solids; and an extract of herb or spice plant solids having a low bacterial count due to the high temperature employed in its production and having improved stability produced according to the process due to edible antioxidant therein; and residual spice or herb plant solid having a low bacterial count due to the high temperature employed in its production and having its tissue ruptured so as to produce quick release of the principal flavor, aroma, colour, or antioxidant component therein, and which is standardized with respect to the principal flavor, aroma, colour, or antioxidant component of interest, produced by the process of the present invention.

The Present Invention

In General

Raw Capsicum or other spice or herb solids, either ground (usually to pass US 40 mesh, and preferably to pass at least US 20 mesh) or unground if coarse particles are desired in the residual solid or cake, *e.g.*, spice solids having a moisture range of about 0.5% to 16% by weight, preferably 0.5 to 12%, and most preferably 1.5% to 10% by weight (ASTA method 2.0), are subjected to a mixing stage, preferably high shear, and in at least one stage an edible solvent is thoroughly dispersed throughout the raw plant material solids.

Typical spice starting plant materials include, for example but without limitation, those of the genus Capsicum including the dried ripe fruits of Capsicum frutescens L. (chilies), Capsicum annum L. (Spanish peppers), Capsicum annum L. var. longum Sendt, its hybrid Louisiana Sport Pepper, and Capsicum chinense (Scotch Bonnet or habenero), all by way of example and not by way of limitation.

Other spices and herbs of interest include those of the family Solanaceae, as stated representatively Capsicums such as paprika, red pepper, and chili, and Lycopersicon, representatively tomato, all containing carotenoid pigments; Umbelliferae, representatively celery, lovage, dill, carrot, cilantro, fennel, cumin, caraway, parsley, angelica, and anise; Compositae, representatively marigold, artemisia, and tarragon; Leguminosae, representatively fenugreek; Labiatae, representatively rosemary, thyme, sage, oregano, marjoram, mint, savoury, and basil; Zingerberacae, representatively ginger, cardamom, and turmeric, Lauraceae, representatively laurel, cinnamon, cassia, and bay; Myrtaceae, representatively allspice and clove; of the genus Myristica, representatively mace and nutmeg; of the genus Piper, representatively black and white pepper; of the genus Vanilla, representatively vanilla; of the genus Allium, representatively onion and garlic; of the genus Sesamum, representatively sesame seed; Cruciferae, representatively mustard and horseradish; the defining characteristic being that it is a spice or herb plant material from which flavor, aroma, colour, and/or antioxidant can be extracted and used to flavor and/or colour foods and beverages or otherwise employed to enhance the palatability of foods and beverages.

The comminuted or uncomminuted plant material is subjected to a plurality of mechanical pressing stages, whereby a concentrated extract of principal components is obtained and a final utilizable and preferably standardized residual solid is produced. The selected edible solvent is introduced into the residual solid at a mixing stage at some point prior to the last pressing stage. The edible solvent, now containing extract, is cycled back to the previous stage, thus always supplying a solvent extract with increasing principal component concentration to the previous mixing and pressing stages. As the extract/edible solvent is passed through each stage countercurrent to the solids flow, a portion of the edible solvent is squeezed or pressed out, thereby extracting a portion of the principal components of interest. As the edible solvent/extract passes countercurrent to the solids, the extracted principal components are progressively concentrated in the extract in a continuous process and the residual principal components end up in the final residual solids known as the cake.

By varying the pressure, temperature, spice solids feed rate, solvent addition rate, and the number of mixing and pressing stages, the concentration of the principal components can be controlled in both the extract and the residual solid.

As will be apparent to one skilled in the art, variations in the process of the present invention can be employed to produce variations in result, the most advantageous of which are the production of both plant material extract of standardized marketable potency and edible residual solid plant material also characterized by standardized marketable potency, and with the edible residual solids also characterized by rapid release of the principal components of interest. Moreover, in the process of the present invention, the spice or herb plant solids have their tissue ruptured so as to provide quick release of the flavor, aroma, colour, or antioxidant component therein when in actual use, *i.e.*, when incorporated into foods or beverages.

For example, using 200 ASTA paprika starting material of about 5% moisture, a 20% soy oil addition, and leaving a residual cake extractable yield of 9.8% by weight of the starting plant solids material, gives an extract with a colour value of 850 ASTA and a residual cake colour value of approximately 50 ASTA. Contrastingly, using a 10% soy oil addition (instead of 20%) yields a cake having about 65 ASTA colour value and, by increasing the residual cake extractable yield to 12.5% by weight of starting plant solids material, the colour value of the residual cake rises to about 100 ASTA and that of the extract to about 1400 ASTA. The lowest colour extract for paprika normally traded is 1,000 ASTA.

Although less than 20% edible oil addition is highly desirable and can be used in many cases, with some edible solvent systems wherein the principal compounds of interest have a limited solubility, or when a more dilute extract and/or lower concentration of principal compounds is desired in the residual solids, more than 20% by weight of edible solvent addition will be required inasmuch as a suitable concentration of principal compounds in the finished extract and in residual solid can in some cases be produced only by the employment of the higher dilution.

Due to the successive treatments of high pressure and pressure relief, with pressures ranging from 6,000 to 30,000 PSI in the pressing stages of the operation, in the presence of added edible solvent, *e.g.*, vegetable oil, and due to frictional heat generated in these high pressure zones, both the residual solid and the extract exiting the process surprisingly have a significantly reduced microbial load over that of the starting material even at moisture levels significantly lower than those indicated by the prior art and, also surprisingly, exhibit increased resistance to oxidative degradation of the carotenoid pigments which are responsible for the characteristic red-yellow colour of various spices, *e.g.*, Capsicums.

The extract from the first or any selected pressing stage may be centrifuged or filtered to provide the finished extract free of particulate solids. Preferably, the fine particulate solids and gums in the extract may be hydrated to about 5% to 200% by weight of the gums and solids prior to centrifugation or filtration to give a crystal clear extract. If water is not used to hydrate the solids and gums, the fine particulate solids from the extract may conveniently be combined with the final residual solids, recycled back into mixing and pressing stages of the process, or alternatively discarded. If water is used to hydrate the solids and gums, it is preferred that the solids and gums be added back to the final residual press solids or discarded.

The edible solvent employed according to the process of the present invention, as illustrated by the following Examples, may be any edible solvent and especially those selected from the group consisting of soybean oil, corn oil, cottonseed oil, rapeseed oil, sesame oil, peanut oil, mon-, di-, and triglycerides, lecithin, essential oils of spices, herbs, or other plants, edible alcohols, propylene glycol, glycerine, hydrogenated or partially hydrogenated fats or oils, limonene, polyoxyethylene sorbitan esters, or any other edible vegetable or animal fat or oil, or mixture thereof, or edible derivatives thereof, the essential aspects of the solvent being that it serves as an extraction aid in which the principal components of the material being extracted are soluble and that it be edible.

The edible solvent, according to the present invention, is combined with the raw material solids to be processed in a proportion of about 5% to about 50% by weight, and frequently amounts as low as 5 to 20% by weight are possible, based on the weight of the starting raw material solids to be extracted. The lower percentages frequently produce a more acceptable and marketable concentration of principal components of interest in both the extract and the residual solids.

The temperature to be employed during the processing and especially in the pressing stages of the process of the invention may be varied widely, but the process is generally carried out at a temperature below about 450° F., and between about 130° F. and 325° F., most preferably above 180° F. and especially between about 180° F. and 235° F.

Temperatures in excess of 130° F. are advantageously employed to achieve acceptable yields and increased throughput rates as compared to the prior art. Higher temperatures are employed to control an increased degree of browning and, most importantly, to reduce the microbial load of both the solids and the extract while at the same time imparting increased resistance to oxidative degradation of the carotenoid pigments of Capsicums in both the extract and the residual solids. Thus, when it is desired that the residual solids from the process have a desirable darkened, caramelized appearance and/or flavor, a reduced microbial load, and increased resistance to oxidation, this is readily attained by increasing the temperature of the solids and the extract during the process, especially during the pressing stages thereof.

When an antioxidant or chelator is introduced into the process for protection of the spice or herb being processed, this is preferably another plant material or an extract thereof, preferably of the Labiatae family, such as rosemary, thyme, or sage, which is known for its protective antioxidant activity (U.S. Pat. No. 5,209,870), or sesame, or tea catechins, but may alternatively be a suitable edible and preferably an approved food grade additive such as ethoxyquin, BHA, BHT, TBHQ, tocopherol, Vitamin C (*e.g.*, as in U.S. Pat. Nos. 5,290,481, 5,296,249, or 5,314,686), citric acid, EDTA, or the like. The process of the present invention is particularly adaptable to the extraction of any spice or herb plant material solids containing carotenoid pigments or other components which provide colour and/or flavor, pungency, aroma, or antioxidant activity, such as present in rosemary, thyme, sage of the Labiatae genus, to a food with which combined.

Detailed Description of the Invention

The following examples are given to illustrate the present invention but are not to be construed as limiting.

Example 1: Paprika Extraction: Dehydrated paprika (5.5% moisture) is ground in a hammer mill and the resulting ground paprika (95% passing US 40 mesh) is admixed with about 10% by weight of soy bean oil and processed in a countercurrent extraction system involving three (3) pressing stages, each using an Egon Keller Model KEK-100 Screw Press, with the extracts from the second and third stages being returned to the preceding mixing stage before being removed from the process at the end of the first press stage.

A high shear, high speed pin mixer or equivalent is used to mix the soy oil or extracts from the second and third press stages into the ground spice or residual solid from the preceding stage. This recycling is continuous.

The raw material paprika solids are continuously fed at a rate of about 240 lbs. per hour with a total contact time in each mixing stage of about 15-60 seconds. The residence time in each press is 5-60 seconds. The pressing stages are operated at about 10,000 PSI internal pressure and about 200 degrees Fahrenheit, which is maintained by cooling with water through the bore of the press shafts.

The starting colour value of the ground paprika solids is 200 ASTA. The principal components extracted and standardized in both the extract and the residual solid are the carotenoid pigments. The resulting final soy-paprika extract has a colour value of about 1,375 ASTA and the reground paprika residual solid from the final (3rd) press stage has a colour value of about 85 ASTA.

Example 1A: Variation: By varying the percentage of edible solvent employed from about 5% to 20%, the pressure from about 6,000 to 30,000 PSI, the number of countercurrent mixing and pressing stages from 2 to 5, with return of the extract from each press stage to the preceding mix stage before final removal from the process in the first press stage, varying the temperature from about 130° F. to 280° F., and removing the seed from the paprika solids prior to grinding, the resulting extract ranges in colour value from about 2,700 ASTA to about 800 ASTA and the residual solids range in colour value from 180 ASTA to 35 ASTA.

By regrinding the residual solids (from the final stage) just as is done with fresh, dehydrated paprika, a product in every way comparable to commercially available ground paprika solids is produced. After filtering or centrifuging off the fine particulate solids, the extract can be directly substituted for commercially available paprika oleoresin in every respect.

By varying the pressing temperature of the process from about 130° F. to 325° F., the hue of the reground residual solid is varied from slightly browned to a dark chocolate brown, demonstrating that the degree of brownness can be controlled by the pressing temperature employed. The degree of "brownness" is measured using a Hunter Labscan Spectrocolorimeter with 0 degree illumination, 45 degree circumferential viewing, illuminant D65, 10 degree observer, Ceilab coordinate system.

The hue of the paprika powder is measured by placing the powder in a 2.5-inch diameter cuvette, shaking gently to ensure even coverage, and measuring through the bottom of the cuvette. The results of the varied operating temperatures of the process are shown in Table. The designation L is indicative of the "lightness" of the sample with the higher numbers being lighter or less browned, and the lower numbers being darker or more browned.

Processing Temperature	*Visual Appearance*	*L* Values*
130° F.	Red	40.18
150° F.	Tan-Red	37.25
200° F.	Light Brown Red	33.22
280° F.	Dark Brown Red	29.16
325° F.	Chocolate Red	22.85

The data clearly demonstrate that the degree of browning can be controlled by varying the press temperature at which the process is conducted. This broadens the applications or uses of the residual solid to include a base for toasted chili powder and as a replacement for browned, caramelized paprika. The residual solid can be substituted for ground paprika or chili powder in many common applications and a separate processing step for browning to a desired degree is not required.

The starting ground paprika solids have an aerobic plate count (Analysis run according to Bacterial Analytical Manual By AOAC, 8th edition, 1995, and ISO-GRID Methods Manual, 3rd edition, 1989) of about 14,000,000. The residual solids exiting the extraction system have a count of about 2,000 to 200,000, with the lower count being achieved at the higher temperatures. This is a significant reduction and makes the residual solids per se suitable for any application where treatment with ethylene oxide or irradiation would normally be required.

Example 1B: Antioxidant Addition: The foregoing example is repeated with all materials and conditions being the same, except that the soybean oil edible solvent is supplemented with an antioxidant blend at a concentration of 3% by weight of the original ground paprika solids. The blend consists of about 29% lecithin, 20% powdered ascorbic acid, 5% citric acid, 15% tocopherol, and 1% rosemary extract (in accordance with Chang and Wu U.S. Pat. No. 5,077,069).

The stability of (1) the resulting extract and (2) the residual solids is compared in each case with an untreated control. In such evaluation, the paprika extracts are plated on flour salt to an extent of 2.4% by weight with a mortar and pestle. Two-gram samples are weighed into 13×100 mm test tubes. The test tubes are stored in a thermostatically-controlled oven at 65° C. Samples are withdrawn periodically, extracted with acetone, and the colour at 460 nm of a standard (%) dilution in acetone is determined spectrophotometrically. In the evaluation of the residual solids, two-gram samples of the reground residual solid are substituted for the flour salt dispersions.

The procedure for the "standard dilution" is as follows: The initial colour of the dispersion is determined by pouring two grams of the original dispersion into a 100-ml flask. Acetone is added up to the 100-ml level. The flask is inverted several times. The flour salt is allowed to settle for five minutes. Then three ml of the dilution is pipetted into a 25-ml flask and diluted up to the 25-ml level. The absorbance is read at 460 nm. The 460 nm colour is determined by the formula: ##EQU1## to translate to ASTA colour, multiply the 460 nm colour by 820.

The colour is plotted against time and the time for 1/3 of the starting colour to fade is reported as the 2/3 life.

This is a highly-reproducible measurement, which is sufficiently accurate to evaluate the effectiveness of the antioxidants and will assist the practitioner to optimize formulations for specific uses.

The final extract from the first press stage of the unprotected or unstabilized process has a colour value of about 1375 ASTA and a 2/3 life of 6.5 hours as compared to a colour value of about 1600 ASTA and a 2/3 life of 63 hours for the extract from the protected material. The colour value of the unprotected or unstabilized residual solids is about 85 ASTA with a 2/3 life of 54 hours, compared to the protected solids which have a colour value of about 95 ASTA and a 2/3 life of 155 hours. This clearly demonstrates that inclusion of antioxidants can improve not only the colour yields from the extraction process but also at the same time improve the colour stability of both the extract and the residual solids.

Other suitable antioxidants (*e.g.*, lecithin, ethoxyquin, butylated hydroxy anisole (BHA), butylated hydroxy toluene (BHT), tertiary butyl hydroxy quinone (TBHQ), sesame, tea catechins, and Labiatae herb antioxidant activity, finely-divided ascorbic acid, tocopherol, citric acid) can be substituted in whole or in part for the specific antioxidant mixture employed with similar desirable colour-protective results, preferably a naturally-occurring antioxidant from an herb of Labiatae family, *e.g.*, rosemary, sage, or thyme, or powdered ascorbic acid.

Example 2: Effect of Varying Operating Temperatures: Dehydrated paprika solids (2.5% moisture) were ground in a hammer mill and the resulting ground paprika (95% passing US 40 mesh) was processed with about 15% by weight of soy bean oil in a countercurrent extraction system as in Example 1 involving two (2) pressing stages, with extracts from the second press stage being returned to the preceding (first) mix stage before being removed from the process at the first press stage.

Upon exiting the first press stage, distilled water was metered continuously into the crude extract at a rate of 75% by weight of the gums and solids by means of an inline static mixer. The weight of the gums and fine particulate solids in the extract was determined by diluting one gram of the crude extract in nine grams of acetone. The mixture was spun down for three minutes at 2000 G's in a laboratory centrifuge. The solids separated were air dried and the weight of the gums and solids was calculated as a percentage of the weight of the starting extract. The hydrated gums and solids removed from the extract were continuously returned to the final residual press solids via a high shear, continuous pin mixer installed immediately following a water-jacketed cooling screw which received the residual solids from the second press stage.

Prior to hydration and centrifugation, the extract contained approximately 10% by weight of gums and fine particulate solids as determined by the above-described method. Following hydration and centrifugation the gums and particulate solids amounted to no more than 1% by weight of the extract and the extract was a crystal clear solution, free of any suspended insoluble materials.

The colour value of the starting ground paprika was about 150 ASTA. The pressing stages were operated at about 20,000 to 30,000 PSI. The extraction process was started with the presses operating at about 80° F. as measured by the temperature of the cake exiting the presses.

The temperature of the presses was controlled by the rate of flow of cooling water through the bore of the press shafts and the screen cages to keep the operating temperatures in the range of 80° to 180° F. Over the time of the extraction run, the operating temperatures of the presses, as measured by the temperature of the cake exiting the presses, was gradually increased to about 255° F. by first slowing and then stopping the flow of cooling water to obtain operating temperatures of 180-200° F., and then by substituting steam for the water in the shaft and cages at gradually increasing pressures to achieve temperatures of 200-255° F. Samples of the extracted oil and press residual solids were pulled at various temperature intervals as the temperatures were increased. Samples of the residual solids were pulled at two points, the first (non-rehydrated) immediately after exiting the cake-cooling screw following the final (second) pressing stage, and the second after the thus-cooled residual press solids were rehydrated to a moisture content of about 10%.

The samples were assayed for ASTA colour, aerobic and anaerobic plate count, and colour stability over time using methods employed in Examples 1A and 1B.

The advantages of operating the process at a temperature above 130° F., as indicated by the temperature of the cake exiting the presses, can clearly be seen. The plate count of both the extract and the cake are progressively reduced as the temperatures are increased. (Tables 2 & 3)

Effect of Increasing Temperatures on the Plate Count of the Extract

Temperature Degree F	*Aerobic Plate Count*	*Anaerobic Plate Count*
80	1,900,000	790,000
130	1,700,000	800,000
150	1,700,000	660,000
170	1,600,000	590,000

Contd...

Temperature Degree F	*Aerobic Plate Count*	*Anaerobic Plate Count*
175	1,500,000	425,000
180	1,300,000	380,000
190	360,000	150,000
200	300,000	200,000
215	240,000	150,000
225	190,000	65,000
235	170,000	32,000
245	69,000	8,600
255	3,800	830

Effect of Increasing Temperatures on the Plate Count of the Press Solids

Temperature Degree F	*Aerobic Plate Count*	*Anaerobic Plate Count*
80	220,000	55,000
130	160,000	35,000
150	160,000	25,000
170	100,000	20,000
175	32,000	15,000
180	80,000	7,400
190	3,500	800
200	9,800	3,400
215	5,800	2,300
225	4,100	500
235	1,900	1,100
245	5,400	100
255	800	100

The efficiency of extraction is dramatically improved as evidenced by the progressively decreasing ASTA values and the progressively decreasing residual extractable yields of the press residual solids. It is apparent that, to achieve residual extractable yields of less than about 20% by weight of the cake, it is necessary to operate the presses at 130° F. or higher.

Moreover, for obvious reasons of efficiency, temperatures above 180° F., and especially between about 180° F. and about 235° F., are greatly preferred.

Press Cake ASTA and Residual Yields at Progressively Increasing Temperatures

Temperature Degree F	*Press Solids ASTA*	*Press Solids Residual Yield*
80	87	28.28%
130	76	16.40%
150	65	15.72%
170	61	15.72%
175	53	12.36%
180	43	13.88%
190	42	10.84%
200	44	10.72%
215	41	9.96%
225	39	9.50%
235	33	9.28%
245	32	9.00%
255	35	9.80%

Most importantly, the stability of the extract is not adversely affected and is in fact increased. The accelerated study was done according to the procedures described in Example 1B with the colours reported as a percent of the starting colour for each respective sample to adjust for the varying colour yields at the respective temperatures. These results demonstrate that the extract produced at higher operating temperatures exhibits increased resistance to oxidative colour deterioration. This is surprising, as explained in the following.

Press Oleoresin (Extract) Stability, Accelerated, 65° C.

Temperature Degree F	*Hour* 2	*Hour* 4	*Hour* 8	*Hour* 12	*Hour* 17
80	94%	88%	81%	73%	62%
130	94%	89%	82%	75%	64%
170	93%	89%	82%	76%	65%

Contd...

Temperature Degree F	*Hour 2*	*Hour 4*	*Hour 8*	*Hour 12*	*Hour 17*
225	94%	90%	82%	78%	67%
235	94%	90%	82%	77%	69%
255	95%	90%	84%	78%	72%

It is commonly believed that lipid-containing systems, when exposed to heat, will exhibit an increased rate of lipid oxidation that, once initiated, will proceed at an ever-increasing rate. (Rancidity and its Measurement in Edible Oils and Snack Foods, A Review, Robards, Kerr, and Patsalides, Analyst, February 1988, Vol 113). In fact, prior art (U.S. Pat. No. 4,681,769) claims a process for counter-current, high pressure extraction of Capsicums at less than 100° F. and less than 500 PSI for the express reason of protecting the extracted oil from oxidation.

To confirm the positive effect of high temperature treatment in more controlled conditions, a forty gram sample of hexane-extracted oleoresin paprika, with no diluents added, was heated in a beaker on a heated stir plate at 100° C. for eight and one-half hours. A control sample which was unheated, a sample pulled from the heated beaker after four hours, and a sample of the material heated for the full eight and one-half hours were dispersed on flour salt to make dispersions of 1.2% oleoresin by weight of flour salt. Two gram-portions of the dispersions were weighed into test tubes and placed in a 65° C. oven. An initial ASTA colour was run on each dispersion and then ASTA colours were run periodically and the results were plotted versus time to determine the relative stability of the heated and unheated samples.

ASTA Values of Heated & Unheated Oleoresin Paprika (Extract) Over Time

	Heated 4		*Heated 8*
Hours	Unheated	@ 100° C.	@ 100° C.
032.5	31.5	26.0	
229.0	29.0	25.8	
426.0	28.0	25.7	

Contd...

	Heated 4		*Heated 8*
624.0	27.0	25.5	
822.5	25.8	25.3	
1021.0	24.5	25.0	
1220.0	23.0	24.8	
1419.0	22.3	24.5	
1618.0	21.8	24.0	
1817.0	21.0	23.5	
2016.0	20.0	23.0	
2215.1	19.0	22.5	
2414.2	18.5	22.1	
2613.4	18.0	21.8	
2812.9	17.5	21.4	
3012.5	17.0	21.0	

The non-rehydrated press residual solids produced in Example 2 exhibit decreased resistance to oxidative colour loss at the press operating temperatures are increased as predicted by prior art (Bennett et al, U.S. Pat. No. 4,681,769).

Stability of Non-Rehydrated Press Solids at Various Press Operating Temperatures, Expressed as Percent of Starting Colour Retained

Temperature	*Week*	*Week*	*Week*
Degree F	2	4	6
80 86.7%	82.2%	85.5%	
13089.6%	85.5%	84.6%	
17073.3%	65.3%	58.1%	
22561.7%	35.8%	32.5%	
24568.2%	31.0%	19.3%	

But, very importantly, it can be seen that the press residual solids which are rehydrated immediately after exiting the second press stage of the process (Example 2) exhibit significantly increased stability relative to the non-rehydrated solids, thus overcoming the claimed disadvantages from operating at temperatures above 100° F. as set forth in U.S. Pat. No. 4,681,769.

Stability of Rehydrated Press Solids at Various Press Operating Temperatures, Expressed as Percent of Starting Colour Retained

Temperature	*Week*	*Week*	*Week*
Degree F	2	4	6
80	90%	92%	91%
130	93%	91%	92%
170	92%	92%	91%
225	94%	93%	91%
245	95%	94%	93%

In fact, after discounting for the effect on pigment stability of increasing residual extractable yields in the press solids obtained at the lower temperatures, the carotenoid pigments in the residual solids would show enhanced stability for a given residual extractable yield. These are surprising and unexpected results and clearly overcome the supposed obstacle of operating at elevated press temperatures and pressures.

It is further surprising that the colour stability of the residual press solids is significantly improved by controlling the water activity (AW) of the solids in ranges above those suggested for the stabilization of lipid-containing systems by extensive studies and particularly by Nelson and Labuza, Water Activity and Food Polymer Science: Implications of State on Arrhenius and WLF Models in Predictina Shelf Life, K. A. Nelson & T. P. Labuza, Journal of Food Engineering 22, 271-289 (1994). Water activity is defined as the ratio of the vapour pressure of water in a food to the vapour pressure of pure water at the same temperature. Prior art suggests that maximum stability of lipid systems should be attained at water activities of about 0.3 with decreasing stability developing as the water activity is increased above this level. In this example we find precisely the inverse effect on stability of the carotenoid pigments for a given water activity.

In order to confirm the effect of high temperatures in the pressing operation, and to confirm the effect of added moisture, a controlled test was performed on a laboratory scale where the effect of levels of extractable yield in the cake could be controlled to eliminate the effect of variable press cake residual yields on the stability of the carotenoids. A 3,000 gram sample of ground paprika solids (175 ASTA, 9.8% extractable yield) was dried in a lab tray dryer at 100° F. for 16 hours to a moisture content of about 2%. One half of this sample was then heated in an oven at 220° F. for twenty minutes to approximate the temperature in a pressing operation according to the invention.

The other unheated sample served as a control. One hundred gram samples of each of the two materials were rehydrated at approximately 1% intervals up to about 12% moisture. The water activity AW of each was determined using a Rotronics Hygroskop DT, model DT2/1-00IV, water activity instrument. Samples were weighed into sealed test tubes, stored at ambient temperatures of about 72° F. in the dark, and the ASTA colours were determined over a period of eighteen weeks to determine the relative rates of colour degradation. The colour retained (as a percentage of the starting colour for each sample to compensate for the effect of colour dilution with the rehydration water) was plotted against time.

Percent Colour Retained of Unheated Ground Paprika at Various Water Activity Ranges

Water Activity Aw	*Week 1*	*Week 5*	*Week 18*
0.15	74%	57%	42%
0.30	50%	45%	12%
0.40	68%	50%	43%
0.60	83%	68%	55%

Percent Colour Retained of Heated Ground Paprika at Various Water Activity Ranges

Water Activity Aw	*Week 1*	*Week 5*	*Week 18*
0.15	66%	56%	41%
0.30	60%	50%	45%
0.40	80%	62%	57%
0.60	98%	82%	78%

It can be seen in Tables 9 & 10 that the stability of the carotenoid pigments follows almost precisely the inverse of the curve predicted by Nelson & Labuza. It can also be seen from these tables that controlled temperature (with concurrent browning) significantly enhances the stability of the carotenoids above a water activity of 0.3 and particularly in the water activity range of 0.4 to 0.6. Water activity ranges higher than 0.6 were not tested as levels marginally higher than this range will support microbial growth which is not acceptable in a dry spice product.

It can be concluded that the stability of the carotenoid pigments found in Capsicums unpredictably does not follow the commonly-accepted and predicted pattern for lipid oxidation with respect to temperature and water activity as suggested in U.S. Pat. No. 4,681,769, or in the cited literature (Nelson and Labuza, Water Activity and Food Polymer Science: Implications of State on Arrhenius and WLF Models in Predicting Shelf Life, K. A. Nelson & T. P. Labuza, Journal of Food Engineering 22, 271-289 (1994); Rancidity and its Measurement in Edible Oils and Snack Foods, A Review, Robards, Kerr, and Patsalides, Analyst, February 1988, Vol 113); describing the stability of lipid systems.

In fact, high temperature treatment, combined with rehydration of the press solids to a water activity above 0.3, preferably of 0.4 to 0.6, significantly improves stability rather than decreases it. This is a very surprising and unpredicted result.

It is well known that the lipid profile of Capsicum and its extracts, without the addition of any diluents, comprises a mixture of saturated and unsaturated fatty acids, 60-70% being unsaturated linoleic and linolenic, Lipid and Antioxidant Content of Red Pepper, Daood, Biacs, et al., Central Food Research Institute, Budapest, Hungary (1989) and The Nature of Fatty Acids and Capsanthin Esters in Paprika, Nawar et al., Journal of Food Science, Vol 36 (1971).

In fact, Daood et al suggest that "...the presence of triglycerides containing high amounts of unsaturated fatty acids may be an important factor contributing to the fading of paprika during processing and storage." The present findings are just the opposite. Without in any way being limited by theoretical considerations, it is hypothesized that the presently-discovered surprising and unpredicted inverse relationship shown (in Tables 9 & 10) between the stability of carotenoid pigments at given water activities is due to the fatty acids in the substrate being Preferentially attacked by the oxidation reaction at the low (from about 0.05 to 0.2 AW) and higher water activity ranges (above 0.3, preferably about 0.4 to 0.6 AW), thus protecting the carotenoids.

At the intermediate water activity ranges (0.2 to 0.4 AW), where the lipids are best protected, the carotenoids are more readily and preferentially attacked and exhibit low resistance to oxidative degradation.

Another controlled test was conducted to demonstrate the effect of different extractable yields in the residual solid press cake. The effect of higher amounts of unsaturated fatty acids is evident from the results illustrated where fresh, refined, bleached, and deodorized soybean oil with no antioxidants was added at various percentages based on the weight of the paprika. The colour over time was compared to the untreated control in an accelerated study at 65° C.

A typical Refined, Bleached, and Deodorized soy oil has a fatty acid composition of 22.3% Oleic (18:1), 51% linoleic (18:2), and 6.8% linolenic (18:3). (Riegel's Handbook of Industrial Chemistry, 9th Edition, pg 278). It can be concluded that higher levels of unsaturated fatty acids, such as oleic, linolenic, and linoleic, which are found in most vegetable oils, will improve the colour stability of the press residual solids.

Levels of extractable yield in the residual solids above about 15-20% by weight of the residual solids is undesirable as the residual Capsicum solids become difficult to handle for most uses and the efficiency of extraction is reduced, *i.e.*, less colour can be removed from the spice as the residual yield is allowed to increase by decreasing either the pressure or temperature employed.

Percent Colour Retained with Varying Amounts of Soy Oil Added to Ground Paprika

Percent Addition	*Hour* 2	*Hour* 4	*Hour* 6	*Hour* 8
0%	65%	59%	52%	50%
5%	90%	83%	74%	72%
10%	92%	84%	75%	74%
15%	94%	87%	80%	78%
20%	96%	91%	83%	81%

It is readily apparent, comparing the results of the controlled test (Tables 9 & 10) on stability of heated vs unheated material, where oil is controlled at a constant level that, at a given added soy oil content in the press residual solids, the colour stability of the residual press solids is significantly improved when the spice, *e.g.*, a Capsicum, has been exposed to higher temperatures.

This conclusion is not readily apparent in the results shown in Table where the amount of residual vegetable oil left in the press residual solids is higher in the low temperature ranges due to the decreased efficiency of the extraction process at lower temperatures. The presence of higher amounts of residual oils there offers some protection which overshadows the increased protective effect at higher temperatures so evident in Tables.

It can therefore be concluded that much, if not all, of the protection offered by operating the presses at temperatures lower than 100° F. (as claimed in U.S. Pat. No. 4,681,769) as compared to temperatures above 100° F. is simply due to the higher residual oil levels (reduced extraction efficiency) and that, for any given residual oil content, and with rehydrated residual solids, the operating temperatures above 130° F. give superior results, not only in an increased extraction efficiency which allows for a continuous, high speed process with increased throughput rates and significantly reduced microbial activity, but most surprisingly in an increased colour stability of both the extract and the residual press solids, particularly when the press solids are rehydrated.

Comparative Example: According to Bennett U.S. Pat. No. 4,681,769,—Low Temperature and Pressure

The press solids residual yield is much higher at temperatures below 100° F. and much higher (28.3% residual yield) than disclosed in U.S. Pat. No. 4,681,769 (10-15% residual yield). In an effort to more closely model the residual yields of 10-15% (oil) in the cake as disclosed in U.S. Pat. No. 4,681,769, the feed rate for this test was set at about 95 pounds per hour, thus allowing more residence time in the press to expel more extract and to reduce the residual yield of the press residual solids to 10-15%.

Various Non-capsicum Spice or Herb Plant Solids

In addition to the foregoing, the following examples show the applicability of the process of the present invention in the production of herb or spice plant extracts and solids having greatly reduced bacterial counts and without the deterioration alleged by the prior art to occur at temperatures above about 100° F., especially at low water contents which are also contraindicated by the prior art, and with the production in each case of residual spice or herb plant solids having its tissue ruptured so as to produce quick release of the flavor, aroma, colour, or antioxidant component therein when in actual use in a food or beverage, thereby greatly increasing the use effectiveness thereof, and both extract and solids produced by the process being readily standardized with respect to the principal flavor, aroma, colour, or antioxidant component of interest.

Example 3: Paprika Extraction and Flavor/Aroma Activation : Paprika is processed in the same manner as given in Examples 1, 1a, 1b, or 2 using a multiple stage, counter-current process with temperatures being in excess of 130° F. with the residual solids being rehydrated to a water activity of 0.6. By adjusting the amount of edible, food grade solvent, and the pressures and temperatures in the pressing stages, the residual cake solids are standardized with respect to ASTA colour value to produce paprika solids with ASTA colour values equivalent to ground paprika commonly used commercially as described in the above examples.

A sample of the residual cake solids at 120 ASTA was reground to pass US 40 mesh and was compared to the starting, unextracted spice, also ground to pass US 40 mesh and rehydrated to a water activity of 0.6, with respect to flavor and aroma intensity. Ten grams each of the residual cake solids and the unextracted spice were thoroughly mixed with 50 grams of flour salt to make a dispersion that would typify a coating for snack foods used to impart a paprika flavor and aroma. Triangle tests were done on the samples.

The samples were coded with random three digit numbers and twelve expert panelists were asked to identify the sample that had the highest paprika flavor and aroma. Twelve of twelve panelists picked the reground residual cake solids as having a more intense paprika aroma. Eight of twelve picked the reground residual cake solids as having a more intense paprika flavor. By statistical analysis (according to methods described in Sensory Evaluation Techniques, Vol II, by Morten Meilgaard, 1987, page 133) this clearly demonstrates that the residual cake solids have more intense paprika aroma and flavor available in a food system as a result of the high pressure, high shear forces and the attendant disruption of the flavor and aroma containing tissue of the spice.

Example 3a: Colour Activation : A sample of 120 ASTA ground residual cake solids was prepared as in Example 3 above. This was compared to a sample of commercially available 120 ASTA paprika with regard to effective colour release into water to model colour release under conditions typical of those used to prepare a marinade or sauce. One (1) gram each of the ground residual cake solids and commercial ground paprika were added to 100 ml of distilled water and stirred for two minutes at ambient temperature.

The slurries were then filtered to remove all particulate solids and the absorbance of each of the solutions was measured spectrophotometrically at 460 nm. The absorbance of the water solution prepared using the residual press solids was 0.566. The absorbance of water solution prepared with the commercial ground paprika was 0.294. This clearly demonstrates that the effective utilization of the colour, and the colour intensity of the model sauce system, were significantly enhanced by the high pressure, high shear, and high temperature of the pressing and extraction process, which ruptures the tissues of the plant solids.

Example 4: Chipotle Extraction and Flavor/Aroma Activation : Chipotle (smoked and dehydrated Jalapeno capsicum pepper) at 4% moisture is ground to pass US 40 mesh and extracted in a two-stage countercurrent pressing operation with the addition of 6% of an edible solvent mixture consisting of 95% soybean oil and 5% decaglycerol tetraoleate (Mazol PGO 104K) by weight of the starting spice in the same manner as described in the above Examples. The principal components of interest in this spice are the flavor (including capsaicinoids which impart the pungent flavor typical of chili peppers) and aroma compounds (including the smokey aroma).

The pungency of the starting ground Chipotle is 35,000 Scoville (ASTA method 21.0). The pungency of the extract is 200,000 Scoville and the pungency of the residual cake solids is 20,000. Both the extract and the residual cake solids have the characteristic smokey aroma of the starting spice. By varying the addition rate of the soybean oil, the concentration of pungent principles is varied in both the extract and the residual solids. For example, using a 12.5% soy oil addition results in an extract with a Scoville pungency of 165,000 and a residual cake solid of 15,000 Scoville. Increasing the soy oil addition to 15% results in an extract of 150,000 Scoville and a residual solid of 7,500 Scoville. This clearly demonstrates that the spice solids can be predictably standardized effectively and efficiently with respect to the principal flavor compounds without the requirement of traditional blending and replating of solvent-extracted oleoresins as described in prior art (U.S. Pat. No. 2,507,084).

The aroma of the residual cake solids is compared to that of the starting unextracted spice using the Triangle method described in Example 3 by dispersing 10 grams of each in 50 grams of flour salt. Six of the twelve panelists can not pick the extracted Chipotle residual solids as being different from the unextracted starting spice, clearly demonstrating that the high pressure, high shear process provides for a ruptured spice residual solid with equivalent aroma intensity even though a portion of the principal components of interest have been removed with the extract.

The starting raw spice has an aerobic plate count of 80,000,000. The plate count of the final extract and residual cake solids are 15,000 and 1,100,000 respectively, again demonstrating that significant reduction in microbial activity can be achieved at such low water contents.

Example 5: Onion Extraction—Flavor and Aroma Activation : Dehydrated, toasted onion powder (Gilroy Foods, Inc. 92700 Toasted Special Onion Powder) was processed in a high pressure extraction system comprising two pressing stages, using Egon Keller Model KEK-100 Screw Presses. Glycerol monooleate containing 10% propylene glycol (Mazol DF300K) was added to the high shear mixing stage prior to the second pressing stage at 25% by weight of the starting spice. The raw material onion was continuously fed at a rate of about 150 lbs per hour with a total contact time in the pressing stages of about 120 seconds. The pressing stage was operated at about 6,000 psi internal pressure and about 190° F., which was maintained by cooling with water through the bore of the press shaft as needed.

The principal components of interest in both the extract and the residual solids are flavor and aroma constituents typical of toasted onion powder. The resulting final extract from the pressing process has the characteristic aroma and flavor profile at a level approximately 4 times the strength of the starting spice as determined by plating the extract on flour salt at varying concentrations and subjecting the resulting dispersions to triangle tests as described in previous examples compared to the unextracted spice. This clearly demonstrates that the flavor and aroma components of the raw spice can be effectively extracted using high pressure, high temperature mechanical pressing.

The residual cake solids are compared to the unextracted spice by dispersing 20 grams of each in 200 ml of salad oil as in Example 3a above, stirring for 5 minutes, and filtering to remove all particulate solids to compare the effectiveness of flavor release into a model salad dressing system. Twelve trained panelists are asked to pick which salad oil has a more intense toasted onion flavor. Twelve of twelve pick the salad oil prepared with the residual cake solids as having superior and more intense toasted onion flavor and aroma. This is a very surprising and unexpected result as a significant portion of the flavor and aroma of the starting spice was removed with the extract.

Without in anyway being limited by theoretical considerations, it is hypothesized that the nature of the edible solvent system used, in combination with the high temperature, high pressure, and high shear forces generated during the processing of the spice, result in a ruptured spice tissue matrix with the flavor and aroma compounds remaining in the residual cake solids being readily soluble in salad oil which otherwise does not readily dissolve the principal components of interest. It is clear that this process provides very significant economic and functional value over prior art.

Example 6: Black Pepper Extraction, Standardization, and Flavor Activation : Black Pepper, ground to pass US 30 mesh, was subjected to a two-stage, countercurrent extraction process as demonstrated in the previous Examples using Triacetin (glycerol triacetate) as the edible solvent at 7% by weight of the starting spice. The temperature of the residual cake solids exiting the pressing stages was maintained at about 215° F.

The piperine content of the starting spice was 11% by ASTA method 12.1. Piperine is responsible for the characteristic pungent flavor of black pepper. The final extract, after filtering to remove the fine particulate solids, had a piperine content of 41.6% and the residual cake solids had a piperine content of 4.1%, typical of commercially-traded grades of black pepper commonly used in food preparation.

An expert panel compared the ground residual cake solids to commercial ground black pepper at 4% piperine. The panelists unanimously picked the residual cake solids as being more pungent, demonstrating that the high pressure, high shear treatment in combination with an edible food solvent provide a surprisingly improved residual spice solid, as compared to an untreated spice having equivalent levels of the principal compound of interest. This presents a clear advantage over prior art.

Example 7: Rosemary Extraction and Standardization of Antioxidants : Ground, dried Rosemary at 6% moisture was processed in accordance with the procedures described in Example 6 but using a medium chain triglyceride based on caprylic/capric fatty acids (Neobee M-5, produced by the Stepan Company) at a level of 40% by weight of the starting spice, with temperatures of the residual cake solids maintained at about 250° F. with cooling water or steam as needed through the bore of the press shafts.

The starting raw material had levels of Carnosol and Carnosic acid, two of the primary antioxidant compounds present in rosemary, of 0.46% and 2.47% respectively, for a total of 2.93% by weight of active compounds. Carnosic acid and Carnosol levels were determined by extracting a sample with a methanolic solution of Bisphenol A (internal standard). The extract therefrom was analyzed by reverse phase HPLC on a C-18 column using a gradient mobile phase of methanol and methanol: aqueous citric acid buffer and UV detection at 280 nm. The method can be calibrated using a pure sample of Carnosic acid and Carnosol.

The final extract, after centrifuging to remove the fine particulate solids, had 0.49% Carnosol and 5.80% Carnosic acid for a total of 6.2% by weight of active compounds or a two-fold increase in concentration from that of the starting spice. The residual cake solids contained 0.21% Carnosol and 0.23% Carnosic Acid for a total of 0.44% by weight active compounds. This represents about 15% of the active compounds found in the starting spice.

This surprisingly demonstrates that, contrary to prior art, the antioxidant compounds can be efficiently extracted in a continuous, high speed, high pressure process with levels of edible solvent considerably below those disclosed by prior art, providing an extract produced by such a process that is clearly superior in levels of antioxidants. Prior art, in particular U.S.

Pat. No. 3,732,111, discloses a method for extraction of Labiatae herbs using prohibitively high ratios of edible solvent in relation to the weight of the starting spice. This necessarily, by simple dilution, results in an extract of low antioxidant concentration that make the extract so weak with respect to the active compounds that it cannot be used in many food systems where the volume of edible solvent in relationship to the compounds of interest is simply too high.

By varying the ratio of edible solvent to ground spice, and the number of countercurrent pressing stages, the levels of active compounds in the extract and residual solids can be controlled in the same manner as described in previous examples.

The starting ground rosemary had an aerobic plate count of 7,000,000. The final extract and residual cake solids had plate counts of 600 and 35,000 respectively. Again, contrary to prior art which suggests that elevated moisture contents and lengthy holding time are necessary, the present process dramatically and rapidly sterilized both the extract and residual solids at such low moisture contents due to the high temperatures, pressures, and shear forces employed.

Example 8: Turmeric Extraction, Standardization, and Sterilization : Using the general procedures as described in the previous Examples, turmeric at 3% moisture and containing 6% curcumin (ASTA method 18.0) was extracted using 10% by weight of Polysorbate 80.RTM., a polyoxyethylene sorbitan ester, in a countercurrent, two-stage pressing operation with the temperature of the residual cake solids being maintained at about 220° F. Curcumin is the pigment responsible for the intense yellow colour of turmeric. The final filtered extract and the residual cake solids are 20% and 3.5% curcumin respectively.

The plate count of the starting spice is about 50,000,000, the final extract 25,000, and the final residual cake solids 1,500,000. Again, contrary to the teachings of prior art, at such low moisture contents.

By varying the amount of edible solvent added prior to the second pressing stage, the levels of curcumin can be accurately and predictably controlled in both the extract and residual cake solids as described in previous examples.

Example 9: Oregano Extraction, Standardization, Activation, and Sterilization : In the same manner as given in previous Examples, ground oregano at 5% moisture is processed in a two-stage, countercurrent extraction process using 10% by weight of soy bean oil. The presses are operated at about 230° F. as measured by the temperature of the cake exiting the pressing stages. The presses are operated at about 20,000 PSI. The plate count of the starting herb is 5,000,000. The plate counts of the final extract and residual cake solids are 800 and 50,000 respectively demonstrating again, contrary to prior art, that the plate counts of spice and herb solids can be significantly reduced at such low moisture contents.

The residual cake solids are compared for flavor strength to the starting ground herb using the method as described in Example 5. Only six of twelve panelists are able to pick the residual cake solids as being less flavourful than the starting ground herb.

Example 10: Other Families and Species of Herb and Spice Plant Materials : In the same general manner as given in previous Examples, other spices and herbs at moisture contents of less than 10% that contain colour, flavor, aroma, or antioxidant principles, are processed and extracted in accord with the method of the present invention.

Such plant materials include, but without limitation, oregano, basil, mint, marjoram, anise, mace, caraway, carrot, garlic, cinnamon, allspice, clove, ginger, cilantro, parsley seed, sesame, cumin, lovage, tarragon, cardamom, fenugreek, mustard, and vanilla, the primary characteristic of such plant materials being that they impart flavor, aroma, colour, or preservative qualities to the food or beverage system in which they are used, and by way of illustration but not by way of limitation, in each case to produce a concentrated extract from the first pressing stage and residual cake solids from the last pressing stage, both standardized with respect to the principal components of interest, both with significantly reduced microbial load, and the residual cake solids having "activated" or quick-releasing principal components of interest in the food or beverage system in which they are used, and for those containing carotenoid pigment, increased stability of the pigment in both the extract and residual cake solids. All this being accomplished under conditions contrary to prior art: without the use of non-edible solvents, low temperatures, and high moisture contents which develop off flavours, aromas, and colours; and without excessive volumes of edible solvents resulting in extracts and residual solids of limited application due to their low content of principal components of interest.

It is thereby seen that an improved countercurrent process for the extraction of spice and herb plant solids using an edible solvent, whereby improved yields of both extract and residual solids are obtained, whereby both the extract and the residual solids have improved stability and freedom from bacterial contamination due to the higher temperatures employed, whereby due to optional advantageous rehydration of residual solids and level of water activity employed an improved stability in the residual solids is attained, whereby an extract in the form of a clear solution can be obtained by removal of gums and particulate solids in the form of their insoluble hydrates, whereby even greater stability can be effected by the employment of edible antioxidants in the solvent utilized, whereby controlled browning of the residual solids may be conveniently effected, and whereby the residual spice or herb plant solids have their tissue ruptured so as to produce quick release of the flavor, aroma, colour, or antioxidant component therein thereby to provide greatly improved use effectiveness, and whereby all products of the process can be conveniently standardized with respect to the principal flavor, aroma, colour, or antioxidant component of interest, all without the expected disadvantages from employing higher temperatures and lower water content as clearly indicated by the prior art, and whereby all of the stated objects of the invention have been accomplished, has been provided.

It is to be understood that the invention is not to be limited to the exact details of operation, or to the exact compositions, methods, procedures, or embodiments shown and described, as obvious modifications and equivalents will be apparent to one skilled in the art, and the invention is therefore to be limited only by the full scope which can be legally accorded to the appended claims.

Aromatherapy

Basic Principles of Aromatherapy

Essential oils are obtained by 2 main methods:

(1). Expression (also called pressing) *i.e.* cold pressed lemon oil.

(2). Distillation, either steam, water or dry.

For oils such as Camphor it is processed three times to produce the three types of oil. The first produces Brown Camphor, the second Yellow Camphor and the third White Camphor.

The other methods for extraction are:

(1). Solvent. This produces a 'Concrete', a 'Resinoid' and an 'Absolute'.

(2). Enfleurage or Pomade. This method for producing Essential oils is not used much any more, as it is an expensive and time consuming process.

A Concrete is obtained through the use of a hydrocarbon solvent to extract the Essential oil from the plant matter. This is used for the Essential oils such as Rose, Jasmine and Ylang Ylang. The Ylang Ylang concrete is approx. 80% Essential oil and 20% wax. Jasmine is approx. 50% Essential oil and 50% wax. A second extraction may also be performed to the plant matter using alcohol which produces an Absolute such as Neroli.

A Resinoid is obtained by the same method, but it is produced from resin based plants such as Amber and Frankincense. A Pomade was obtained by the use of layers of fat onto which the petals of plants such as Tuberose and Jasmine were laid out and left to dry. The fat collected the Essential oils which were later extracted. This process has now been replaced by solvent extraction.

Essential oils are found in very small quantities in many plants. For example: for every 100 kg of plant matter the following plants produce these amounts of oil:

Eucalyptus	-	3kg
Lavender	-	1.9kg
Ylang Ylang	-	1.6-2kg
Juniper	-	1/2-1.2kg
Rose	-	0.05kg

As you can see it takes a lot of plants to make a small amount of Essential oil.

Plants from different areas/countries can be more expensive (lower % of oil per plant) or cheaper (higher % of oil per plant).

Essential oils are categorized by:

(a) Their plant type *i.e.* Citrus

(b) By their Note. *i.e.* Base note

The plant types are: Citrus, floral, herb, spice, wood and resin. Although the oils can blend with any other oils, they blend better with oils of their own group, or with an oil of a similar group. *i.e.* Lemon (citrus) & Lavender (floral) and Cedarwood (wood) & Patchouli (herb).

The note types are: Top, Middle and Base. Top note oils such as Neroli and Lemon evaporate and lose their aroma quickly when left open. A top note oil will last approx. 1 week if left opened. A middle note oil such as Lavender and Geranium is slightly more stable and will evaporate and lose its aroma approx. 2-3 weeks when left opened. Base note oils are the heavy oils such as Sandalwood and Patchouli which will evaporate much more slowly, taking about a month.

When you smell a blended oil you can usually pick which oils are the top, middle and base oils as the first one you notice will be a top note. The next scent you notice will be from the middle notes and the heavy, lingering scent will belong to the base note. In this way you can tell which oil is which note.

A good blend will contain at least one of each note, to add a layered effect to the blend.

Synthetic Vs. Natural Oils

Most of you will have seen cheap bottles of 'fragrant' oils or bottles of 'blended Essential oils' as well as bottles of 'Pure Essential oils'. Each one has it's own uses.

Fragrant Oils: These are the synthetic oils.

Scientists have been able to reproduce about 90% of the natural occurring Essential oil. This is what a fragrant oil is. It is the remaining 10% of the natural Essential oil that holds the therapeutic content of the oil, and that 10% is what distinguishes the two.

Fragrant oils have NO therapeutic content, they smell nice (sometimes better than the Essential oils!) but that is all that they should be used for. They work well in oil burners, in baths, in pot pourri, as a perfume and various other uses, but will have no healing effect other than to smell nice.

Blended Essential Oils: These are made from Pure Essential oils, but have been diluted with a 'Carrier oil', usually Sweet Almond, jojoba, Safflower or Apricot Kernel.

These oils are blended because Essential oils are too strong to apply directly to the skin, they must be diluted first. The Blended oil has been diluted so it is safe to apply directly onto the skin. These have therapeutic qualities, which are usually printed on the label.

They may also be blended to make them cheaper, such as Rose, Neroli, Jasmine, Chamomile and Ylang Ylang

Pure Essential Oils: These are the Essential oils in their 100% pure state.

These oils should never be applied straight onto the skin, and many Essential oils will have safety data printed onto the label if they have any harmful effects. (there are a few exceptions to the "never put oils directly on the skin" rule... which I will go into later) When purchasing an Essential oil there are 4 ways to help tell if you are buying the pure oil:

(1) Look for the words "100%" and "Pure Essential oil". This is only a guide as many brands of fragrant oil have 100% pure written on them, and some brands of Essential oils

(such as the brand I use) don't have 100% pure on the label. There are also sneaky people who use the "100% Pure Essential Oil" as their brand name....(and if the word 'fragrant' appears anywhere, chances are it isn't an Essential oil.)

(2) Smell the oils, Pure Essential oils smell like the plant it comes from. If the scent is slightly fake, very sweet or in the case of Rose really strong, it is more likely to be a fragrant oil.

(3) Look at the price, Pure Essential oils are expensive, due to the quantity of plants needed to produce the oil (for *e.g.* it takes approx. 15 roses to make 1 drop of Rose oil.) Each oil should have a different price, as some are cheaper to produce than others. As a general rule... if they are under $5 (Australian money... not sure of the prices in other countries) they are probably either blended or a fragrant oil.

(4) There are no Essential oils of Strawberry, Dewberry, Rainforest or Nanna's Garden. If something like these is packaged the same and on the same stand, then chances are all the oils are synthetic oils.

This is a guide only... but it helps to work out which ones are "fake" and which ones are "real". The store keeper may not know the difference, as they buy products from a distributor, and many haven't a clue what they are... they just know they sell well:

Aromatherapy Vs. "Normal" Medicine

Many people take Aspirin for headaches although many tests have proven that Aspirin can cause stomach upsets, thin the blood, cause liver damage and contribute to anaemia. Yet people take many of these a day to relieve headaches, and think they are safe.

Antibiotics are used for infections because they kill bacteria. However there are good bacteria living in our bodies, without which our bodies can not work efficiently. Antibiotics kill off all bacteria, and many people suffer from thrush and other illnesses as a result. The other concern with antibiotics is that each time they are used, the body builds up a resistance to them, much the same way our bodies build up a resistance to the Smallpox or Measles virus when we are vaccinated. Stronger doses of antibiotics are then needed to fight the infections, and the circle continues.

Aromatherapy works on the wholistic approach. It treats the whole body at the one time. Aromatherapy has no negative side effects when used properly, and is non- addictive.

Aromatherapy Explained (Simply)

People think of Aromatherapy as being smell therapy, but this isn't the case. The essential oils can used in many different methods, I will be explaining those later... but the reason people think of them as being smell therapy, is that the blood vessels in your nose are very close the surface of your skin....so the molecules of "healing goodness" can be absorbed into the body quickly (and they do smell nice...well....some of them!) the healing effects can also pass through the skin anywhere on your body, and enter the blood stream, where they work on the troubled areas of the body.

Essential oils, unlike prescription drugs, work only on those areas that are "broken" *i.e.* they do not go into healthy tissues, and start working there... they travel around your body, and look for the illnesses, and target them, leaving the rest of your body alone. It is because of this, that if you run lavender oil into your fingertip, it will help your infected toe...even though the oil never touches the actual toe. (and your headache, and cut finger!!!).

Using Essential Oils

There are 8 main ways to use the Essential oils, they are as follows:

Inhalation:

(1). Straight from the bottle—Headache, memory booster, nausea etc.

(2). Oil burner—Kill airborne bacteria (prevents colds spreading to others), insomnia, stress etc. Put 3-5 drops in a water filled well of the oil burner, and replace as needed. NEVER burn Essential oils without water... it damages them

(3). Drops on a tissue (carry with you or place under pillow etc.)—colds, coughs, migraine etc. 1-2 drops on a tissue will be ample

(4). Drops in sink/bowl of hot water—colds, respiratory infection, catarrh (runny nose) etc. stick your head over the sink/bowl, with eyes closed and inhale the vapour. No more than 5 drops to half a sink full of water (which is all you need)

Bat:

(1). Hot/warm bath—colds, muscle cramp, stiffness etc. 10 drops Maximum

(2). Cold bath—Fever. 10 drops Maximum

(3). Foot bath—Athlete's foot, blisters, aching feet etc. Use a bucket or bowl big enough to comfortably put your feet in. 5 drops Maximum

(4). Shallow bath—Thrush, Piles etc. a bath deep enough to cover the problem area. 5 drops maximum

If using peppermint oil, you may want to use only half the recommend drops.... as my Aromatherapy teacher said "It runs amok amongst your genitals" it has a cooling effect that you may not wish to have touching sensitive areas.

You will need to swish the water around. There is a product called Solubalizer that may be useful. It makes the oil dissolve in water, although the same effect can be to mix the oil with isopropyl alcohol (rubbing alcohol) or vodka, which will make it water soluble. 5 drops to 1tsp alcohol. I have also heard that the same effect can be achieved with milk, but I am not sure.

Massage:

(1). Massage diluted oil onto effected area - varicose veins, strains, constipation Muscle aches etc.

(2). Massage diluted oil all over body - Stress, insomnia, anxiety etc.

Both, use a 3% dilution for normal skin, 1% for face or sensitive skin (explained further below).

Internally: Most Essential oils are toxic and should NEVER be taken internally. It is safest to assume that ALL Essential oils are toxic and therefore none should be taken internally.

Many Aromatherapy books suggest a mouth wash or a gargle for gum problems or throat infections, however it is dangerous and other methods work just as well. There are many different species of the same oil, for example Birch has 2 varieties, white and sweet. White birch is non-toxic, but sweet birch is fatally toxic. I would not use ANY Essential oils internally, especially in their pure state, as there are many other methods of application which are much safer. {as I was saying in a previous section, even rubbing an oil on your toe will help a sore throat, so it isn't worth ingesting something that is potentially harmful, although I have gargled with 2 drops Bergamot oil mixed with a cup of warm water}

Directly To The Skin: There are only four Essential oils which may safely be applied directly onto the skin an all should have a patch test done first. All essential oils are acidic, have you ever seen what they do to plastic?

Place a drop of the oil onto the back of your wrist, cover with a Band-Aid and leave for 1 hour. If no irritation has occurred you may use it. If irritation does occur, bathe the area in cool water and dilute the oil with a carrier oil. Only the four Essential oils listed below may be applied to skin directly, and only onto an effected area *i.e.* a cut or burn. Do not use as a massage oil, or slather it all over your skin:

Lavender, Sandalwood, Tea tree and some say Lemon, ylang ylang or Chamomile.

There is no need to apply any essential oil directly onto the skin, an essential oil blended 3% into a carrier oil will have exactly the same healing properties as a full strength oil... so not only do you run the risk of burning the skin by applying them neat, you are also wasting oil:)—Scrooge McObsidian here:)

(1). Drops of oil in cold water for cold compress - fever, swelling etc.

(2). Drops of oil in hot water for hot compress - Headache, period pain etc.

To make a compress, half fill a bowl or sink of either hot or cold water, and add 3-5 drops of essential oil.... soak the cloth in this water for a few moments, wring out, and apply to the effected area.

Perfume:

(1). Use same dilution as massage oil, use a carrier oil of Apricot kernel or other light oil. Dab behind ears, wrists etc.

Skin/Hair Tonic:

(1). Use this when an oil is not suitable, for example on an oily scalp, or to dry out a cut. use 5 drops essential oil into a teaspoon of Isopropyl alcohol (rubbing alcohol) or vodka

Dilutions:

Babies 0-12 months—1 drop of Rose or Lavender or chamomile in 1 teaspoon of carrier oil, or in a bath.

Infants 1-5 years - 2-3 drops of Rose, Lavender, Chamomile, Sandalwood, Tangerine, Ylang Ylang or Neroli in 1 teaspoon of carrier oil or in a bath.

Children 6-12 years -Use as for adults, but half the concentration.

3% dilution:

For 100 mls of carrier oil use 60 drops of Essential oil.

For 25 mls of carrier oil use 15 drops of Essential oil.

For 5 mls of carrier oil (1 teaspoon) use 3 drops of Essential oil.

1% dilution:

For 100 mls of carrier oil use 20 drops of Essential oil.

For 25 mls of carrier oil use 5 drops of Essential oil.

For 5 mls of carrier oil (1 tsp) use 1 drop of Essential oil.

For normal use do not exceed 3% Essential oil dilution.

For use on face or other sensitive skin use a 1% Essential oil dilution.

Pregnancy - use half the dilution and none of the contraindicated oils.

Contraindications

Aromatherapy oils are concentrated and should not be applied to the skin or taken internally. There are also other times when Essential oils should be treated with caution or not be used at all, these are called Contraindications. The following is a list of the contraindications for the various Essential oils.

Oils not to be Used at All: These oils are dangerous for anyone except a qualified Aromatherapist to use. They are either extremely toxic or cause severe skin irritation even in a diluted state. These oils are:

Bitter Almond, Arnica, Boldo, Broom, Buchu, Calamus, Camphor (brown & Yellow), Cassia, Chervil, Cinnamon (bark), Costus, Deertongue, Elecampane, Fennel (bitter), Horseradish, Jaborandi, Melilotus, Mugwort, Mustard, Oregano, Pennyroyal, Pine (dwarf), Rue, Sage (common), Santolina, Sassafras, Savine, Savoury, Tansy, Thuja, Thyme (red), Tonka, Wintergreen, Wormseed and Wormwood.

Oils that should be Used in Small Doses for no Longer Than 2 Weeks: These oils are fairly toxic or may have side effects such as nausea, vomiting and headaches and should be used with extreme caution:

Ajowan, Anise star, Aniseed, Basil (exotic), Bay laurel, Bay (west indian) Calamintha, Camphor (white), Cascarrilla bark, Cassie, Cedarwood (virginian), Cinnamon (leaf & bark), Clove (bud), Coriander, Eucalyptus, Fennel (sweet), Hops, Hyssop, Juniper, Nutmeg, Parsley, Pepper (black), Pine, Sage (spanish), Tagetes, Tarragon, Thyme (white), Tuberose, Tumeric, Turpentine and Valerian.

Oils that Irritate the Skin if Used in High Concentration: These oils should be used in half the recommended dilution, and no more than 3 drops in a bath. These oils are:

Ajowan, Allspice, Aniseed, Basil (sweet) Black pepper, Borneol, Cajeput, Caraway, Cedarwood (Virginian), Cinnamon (leaf), Clove (bud), Cornmint, Eucalyptus, Garlic, Ginger, Lemon,

Parsley, peppermint, Pine (needle, Scotch & Longleaf), Thyme (white) and Tumeric.

Oils that Cause Irritation on Sensitive Skin: These oils may cause eczema or dermatitis with people who have very sensitive skin. (For people with senstive skin always test the oil on the back of your wrist, and leave for an hour. If irritation occurs bathe area with cold water and try a weaker concentration.) These oils are:

Aniseed, Basil (french), Bay laurel, Benzoin, Bergamot, Cade, Cajeput, Cananga, cedarwood (virginian), Chamomile (Roman and German), Citronella, Garlic, Geranium, Ginger, Hops, Jasmine, Lemon, Lemongrass, Lemon balm (Melissa), Litsea cubeba, Loveage, Mastic, Mint (pepper & spear), Orange, Peru balsam, Pine (scotch & longleaf), Styrax, Tea tree, Thyme (white), Tolu balsam, Tumeric, Turpentine, Valerian, Vanilla, Verbena, Violet, Yarrow and Ylang Ylang.

Oils that are Phototoxic: These are oils which can cause the skin to darken if exposed to direct sunlight. Do not use these oils at all if the area will be exposed to sunlight. These oils are:

Angelica root, Bergamot, Cumin, Ginger, Lemon, Lime, Loveage, Mandarin, Orange and Verbena.

Oils that should be Avoided during Pregnancy: Due to the effects of these oils on the reproductive organs, and the sensitivity of the foetus, certain oils should not be used at all during pregnancy. These oils are:

Ajowan, Anjelica, Anise star, Aniseed, Basil, Bay laurel, Calamintha, Cedarwood (all types), Celery seed, Cinnamon (leaf), Citronella, Clary sage, Clove, Cumin, Cypress, Fennel (sweet), Hyssop, Jasmine, Juniper, Labdanum, lovage, Marjoram, Myrrh, Nutmeg, Parsley, Penyroyal, Peppermint, Rose, Rosemary, Snakeroot, sage, Tarragon and Thyme (white)

Oils that should be Avoided with High Blood Pressure: These oils should not be used:

Black pepper, Hyssop, Lemon, Lemongrass, Nutmeg, Rosemary, Sage (spanish & Common) and Thyme.

Oils that should be avoided with low blood pressure. These oils should not be used:

Chamomile (Roman & German), Lemon balm, Lavender (true), Marjoram (sweet) and Ylang ylang.

The oil that should be avoided for diabetes. Anjelica.

The oil that should be avoided for kidney problems. Juniper.

Oils that should be not be Used with Homeopathic Treatments: These oils are not to be used by anyone receiving homeopathic treatment:

Black pepper, camphor, eucalyptus and peppermint.

Oils that should be Avoided with Alcohol Consumption: These oils will increase the effects of alcohol:

Aniseed, clary sage and fennel.

The oil that should be avoided with depression. Basil.

Oils that should be Avoided with Epilepsy: These oils should not be used:

Fennel, Hyssop, Sage and Rosemary.

The Common Essential Oils

The following information has been gathered from many books over many years. Some oils work by promoting balance, which is why they are listed as working well with things such as oily skin and dry skin. What this means is that if your skin is oily, it will help dry it out, if it is dry it will help add moisture. In other words, it will balance.

Different sources will give different properties to the Essential oils - some may even contradict others. It is for this reason that it is best to leave Aromatherapy to trained professionals.

The following information is not intended to prescribe or diagnose in any way. It is not meant to be a substitute for professional medical advice/assistance. The intention of this list is to give information on the historical usage of Aromatherapy. Please consult your doctor or other health professional if you have any medical complaints. Do not attempt to self diagnose or self prescribe herbal treatments for yourself or others. The Author (Obsidian) shall not be responsible for any misuse or abuse of this information.

Aniseed

Botanical Name: Pimpinella Anisum

Note - Top to middle

Type - Spice

Family - Umbelliferae

Part - Herbs/seeds

Extraction - Steam Distillation

Aroma: Sweet and spicy, pungent, Licorice like, very warming.

Blends well With: Amyris, Bay, Cardamon, Caraway, Cedarwood, Coriander, Dill, Fennel, Galbanum, Mandarin, Petitgrain, Rose wood.

Contraindications: Sensitive skin, Pregnancy, Over use can cause sluggishness, drowsiness and dizziness. In extreme cases can cause cerebral congestion and circulatory problems.

Properties: Carminative, Antiseptic, Antispasmodic, Decongestant, Parasiticide, Antiemetic, Aphrodisiac, Cardiac, Digestive aid, Diuretic, Expectorant, Galactagogue, Insecticide, Laxative, Parturient, Pectoral stimulant, Stomachic.

Uses: Respiratory problems, Digestive problems, Flatulence, Indigestion, Period pains, Stimulate lactation, Lice, Scabies, Muscular aches and pains, Rheumatism, Bronchitis, Coughs, Colic, Cramp, Colds, Stimulate the mind, Dyspepsia, Nausea, Vomiting, Stimulating peristalsis, Oliguria (low quantity of urine), Stimulates cardiac fatigue, Lice, Scabies, Infectious skin diseases.

Cautions: Not generally recommended for use in the home as prolonged or over use may be harmful.

Basil (Sweet)

Botanical Name: Omicum Basilicum

Note - top

Type - Herb

Family - Labiatae

Part - Flowering top

Extraction - Steam Distillation

Aroma: Very clear, sweet and slightly spicy.

Blends well With: Bergamot, Black pepper, Citronella, Chamomile, Clary Sage, Geranium, Hyssop, Lavender, Lemongrass, Lime, Marjoram, Melissa, Neroli, Peppermint, Rose, Sandalwood, Verbena.

Contraindications: Pregnancy, Sensitive skin, Do not use to excess.

Properties: Soothing, Uplifting, Antiseptic, Insect repellent, Digestive aid, Antispasmodic, Emmenagogue, Analgesic, Antidepressant, Antispasmodic, Antivenomous, Aphrodisiac, Bactericide, Carminative, Cephallic, Expectorant, Febrifuge, Galactagogue, Insecticide, Nervine, Stomachic, Sudorific, Tonic, Restorative, Stimulant, Vermifuge, Effects adrenal cortex, Imitates oestrogen, Minimise uric acid in muscles, stimulates blood flow, Helps expel afterbirth, Cleanse intestines and kidneys.

Uses: Fatigue, Depression, Respiratory infections, Colds, Cough, Bronchitis, Asthma, Sinusitis, Fever, Gout, Indigestion, Insect bites and stings, Breast engorgement, Fainting, Flatulence, Insomnia, Muscular aches and pains, Rheumatism, Anxiety, Migraine, Nervous tension, Sharpening senses, Nerve tonic, Concentration, Hysteria, Headaches, Temporary paralysis, Nasal polyps, Earache, Allergies, Bronchitis, Emphysema, Flu, Whooping cough, Catarrh, Vomiting, Gastric spasm, Nausea, Dyspepsia, Hiccups, Menstrual problems, Scanty periods, Fertility problems, Fatigue, Stress, Poor circulation.

Bay

Botanical Name: Laurus Nobilis

Note - top

Type - Spice

Family - Lauraceae

Part - Leaves and twigs

Extraction - Steam Distillation

Aroma: Sweet and spicy, similar to Cinnamon

Blends well With: Citrus Oils, Cedarwood, Clary Sage, Coriander, Cypress, Eucalyptus, Ginger, Hyssop, Juniper, Lavender, Lemon, Marjoram, Myrtle, Orange, Rose, Rosemary, Thyme, Ylang Ylang.

Contraindications: Sensitive skin, Pregnancy, Irritate mucous membranes.

Properties: Analgesic, Antineuralgic, Antiseptic, antispasmodic, Aperitif, Astringent, Cholagogue, Diuretic, Emmenagogue, Febrifuge, Hepatic, Insecticides, Parturient, Stimulant, Stomachic, Sudorific, Tonic, Mildly narcotic, Warms emotions, Reproductive tonic, Uplifting.

Uses: Colds, Flu, Bronchitis, Digestive aid, Dyspepsia, Flatulence, Appetite stimulant, Settles stomach, Liver and Kidney tonic, Rheumatism, Aches and pains, Sprains, Fever, Infectious disease, Scanty periods, Speeds up childbirth, Ear infections, Dizziness, Restores balance, Minor respiratory problems, Indigestion.

Cautions: People prone to sensitive or allergy prone skin should not use Bay oil. Use in moderation and never undiluted.

Bergamot

Botanical Name: Citrus Bergamia

Note - top

Type - Citrus

Family - Rutacaea

Part - Peel

Extraction - Expression

Aroma: Light, delicate, refreshing, something like Orange and lemon with slight floral undertones.

Blends well With: Basil, Cardamon, Chamomile, Coriander, Cypress, Eucalyptus, Geranium, Juniper, Jasmine, Lavender, Lemon, Marjoram, Mimosa, Myrtle, Neroli, Palmarosa, Patchouli, Petitgrain, Sandalwood, Ylang ylang.

Contraindications: Phototoxic, sensitive skin.

Properties: Antiseptic, Parasiticide, Antidepressant, Analgesic, Antispasmodic, Carminative, Cicatrisant, Cordial, Deodorant, Digestive, Expectorant, Febrifuge, Insecticide, Sedative, Stomachic, Tonic, Vermifuge, Vulnerary, Keeps pets away from plants, Uplifting, Vitalising, Anti-inflammatory,

Uses: Dandruff, Urinary and Respiratory infections, Skin infections, Throat and mouth infections, Scalp and skin, Psoriasis, Acne, Ulcers, Stress related conditions, Depression, Coldsores, Shingles, Insomnia, Anxiety, Stress, Bad breath, Deodorant, Worms, Intestinal parasites, Colic, Appetite stimulant, Vaginal infections, Flatulence, Boils, Eczema, Varicose Ulcers, Wounds, Tonsillitis, Colds, Fever, Flu, Abscesses, Cystitis, Digestive aid, Eczema, Insect repellent, Oily skin, Infectious diseases, PMS, Dyspepsia, Flatulence, Colic, Indigestion, Gallstones, Anorexia, Breathing difficulties, TB, Chickenpox, Uterine Tonic, STDs, Gastro-intestinal spasm, Cellulite, Sore throat, Bronchitis.

Black Pepper

Note - Middle

Type - Spice

Family - Piperaceae

Part - fruit

Extraction -Distillation

Aroma: Sharp and Spicy

Blends well With: Basil, Bergamot, Cedarwood, Cypress, Frankincense, Geranium, Grapefruit, Juniper, Lemon, Marjoram, Palmarosa, Rosemary, Sandalwood, Ylang Ylang.

Contraindications: Kidney Problems, Sensitive Skin

Properties: Analgesic, Antiemetic, Antiseptic, Antispasmodic, Aphrodisiac, Cardiac, Carminative, Detoxicant, Digestive, Diuretic, Febrifuge, Laxative, Rubefacient, Stimulant, Stomachic, Tonic, Helps frustration, Warms the heart with there is indifference, Dilates local blood vessels, Stimulates peristalsis, Stimulates circulation, Helps form new blood cells, Antidote for fish and mushroom poisoning, Reduces fat,

Increases flow of Saliva, Stimulates appetite, Expels wind, Fortifying stomach, Expels toxins.

Uses: Muscle aches and pains, Tired and aching limbs, Muscle stiffness, Rheumatoid Arthritis, Temporary Paralysis, Vomiting, Bowel problems, Anaemia, Respiratory illnesses, Fever (Small amounts)

Cajuput

Note - top

Type - Herb

Family - Myrtacaea

Part - leaves and twigs

Extraction - Distillation

Aroma: Sweet, herbaceous and rather penetrating

Blends well With: Angelica, Bergamot, Birch, Cardamon, Cedarwood, Clove, Eucalyptus, Geranium, Immortelle, Lavender, Myrtle, Niaouli, Nutmeg, Pine, Rose, Rose wood, Thyme

Contraindications: Use with caution, sensitive skin, irritate mucous membranes

Properties:Analgesic, Antidontalgic, Antineuralgic, Antirheumatic, Antiseptic, Antispasmodic, Balsamic, Cicatrisant, Decongestant, Expectorant, Febrifuge, Insecticide, Pectoral, Stimulant, Sudorific, Vermifuge, Clears the mind, Balances mind and body, Imitates Oestrogen.

Uses: Respiratory tract infections, Fever, Colds, Pharyngitis, Laryngitis, Bronchitis, Asthma, Ease Chronic Pulmonary Disease, Colic, Inflammation of the intestines, Enteritis, Dysentery, Gastric spasm, Nervous vomiting, Intestinal Parasites, Urinary infections, Cystitis, Urethritis, Neuralgia, Headaches, Toothache, Earache, Gout, Chronic rheumatism, Muscle Stiffness, Muscle aches and pains, Menopausal problems.

Cedarwood

Note - Base

Type - Wood

Family - Cupressacae / Pinaceae

Part - Wood

Extraction - Distillation

Aroma: Woody, reminiscent of sandalwood but slightly "drier" and almost pine tones

Blends well With: Benzoin, Bergamot, Black pepper, Cajuput, Cinnamon, Cypress, Frankincense, Ginger, Jasmine, Juniper, Lavender, Lemon, Linden, Myrrh, Neroli, Patchouli, Pine, Rose, Rosemary, Sandalwood, Vetiver, Ylang Ylang.

Contraindications: Sensitive Skin, Pregnancy.

Properties: Calming, Soothing, Antiseptic, Astringent, Diuretic, Emollient, Expectorant, Fungicide, Insecticide, Sedative, Tonic, Better for chronic (long standing) problems than acute (recent) ones, Balances body and mind, Insect repellent, Aphrodisiac.

Uses: Nervous Tension, Anxiety, Meditation, Bronchitis, Coughs, Catarrh, Excess phlegm, Cystitis, Genito-Urinary tract problems, Kidney problems, Rheumatism, Arthritis, Oily skin, Acne, Clearing scabs, Dermatitis, Psoriasis, Hair tonic, Seborrhoea, Dandruff, Alopecia, Softening skin (especially when mixed with Cypress and Frankincense), Respiratory infections, Glandular problems, Stress, Insect bites and stings, Dermatitis, Eczema, Itching, Coughs, Fungal infections, Hair loss, Ulcers, Bronchitis, Catarrh, PMT, Tiredness, Vaginal infections, Urinary tract infections, Congestion, Sinusitis.

Chamomile

Note -Middle

Type - Flower

Family - Compositae

Part - Flowers

Extraction - Distillation

Aroma: Fruity, apple-like.

Blends well With: Angelica, Basil, Benzoin, Bergamot, Clary sage, Geranium, Jasmine, Lavender, Lemon, Marjoram, Neroli, Palmarosa, Patchouli, Rose, Star Anise, Ylang Ylang.

Contraindications: Pregnancy (early Months)

Properties: Emmenagogue, Analgesic, Antiallergenic, Anticonvulsive, Antidepressant, Antibacterial, Antiemetic, Antiphlogistic, Antipruritic, Antirheumatic, Antiseptic, antispasmodic, Carminative, Cholagogue, Cicatrisant, Digestive, Diuretic, Emollient, Febrifuge, Hepatic, Nervine, Sedative, Splenetic, Stomachic, Sudorific, Tonic, Vermifuge, Vulnerary, Soothing, Calms the mind, Regulates menstruation, Stimulates growth of white corpuscles.

Uses: Anxiety, Tension, Anger, Fear, Promotes relaxation, Gives patience and peace, Allay worry, Insomnia, Muscular pain, Lower back pain, Headache, Neuralgia, Toothache, Earache, Menstrual problems, Period pain, PMT, Menopause, Soothes stomach, Gastritis, Diarrhoea, Colitis, Peptic Ulcers, Vomiting, Flatulence, Irritated bowels, Liver problems, Jaundice, Genito-urinary problems, Anaemia, Burns, Blisters, Inflamed wounds, Ulcers, Boils, Dermatitis, Acne, Herpes, Psoriasis, Broken Capillaries, Improves skin elasticity, Itching, Puffiness, Strengthen tissues, Skin cleanser, Hair tonic, Cramps, Nappy Rash, Nervous Tension, Neuralgia, Bleaching hair, Cracked nipples, Children's tantrums, Fevers, Insomnia, Mastitis.

Cinnamon

Note - Base

Type - Spice

Family - Lauracaea

Part - Bud/Bark/leaf

Extraction - Distillation

Aroma: Spicy, Sharp, Sweet and Musky

Blends well With:Benzoin, Cardamon, Clove, Coriander, Eucalyptus, Frankincense, Galbanum, Ginger, Grapefruit, Lavender, Lemon, Mandarin, Orange, Pie, Rosemary, Thyme.

Contraindications: (Leaf is safer as Bud and Bark can irritate skin more) Use with care in small doses, Pregnancy, High doses could cause convulsions

Properties: Anaesthetic, Antidontalgic, Antiseptic, Antiputrefative, Antispasmodic, Aphridesiac, Astringent, Cardiac, Carminative, Emmenagogue, Escharotic, Haemostatic, Insecticide, parasiticide, Sialogue, Stimulant, Stomachic, Vermifuge, Stimulates tears, Stimulates saliva and mucous, Stimulates secretion of gastric juices, Stimulates Circulatory system.

Uses: Respiratory infections, Colds, Flu, Breathing difficulty, Fainting, Infectious diseases, Viral infections, Intestinal infections, Digestive spasm, Asthenia, Dyspepsia, Colitis, Flatulence, Gastralgia, Diarrhoea, Nausea, Vomiting, Cholera, Typhoid, Period pain, Scanty menstruation, Leucorrhoea, Impotence, Muscle spasm, Rheumatism, Insect bites, Respiratory and digestive problems, Lice, Scabies, Tooth and Gum care, Warts, Wasp stings, Poor circulation, Rheumatism, Anorexia, Colitis, Aids childbirth, Frigidity, Cough, Depression, Flu.

Citronella

Note - Top

Type - Citrus

Family - Graminae

Part - Grass

Extraction - Distillation

Aroma: Sweet and Lemony

Blends well With: Bergamot, Cajuput, Cedarwood, Eucalyptus, Geranium, Lavender, Lemon, Mandarin, Neroli, Orange, Peppermint, Petitgrain, Pine, Sage, Ylang Ylang.

Contraindications: May irritate Sensitive Skin, Pregnancy.

Properties: Antidepressant, Antiseptic, Deodorant, Insecticide, Parasiticide, Tonic for heart and nervous system, Stimulant, Clearing mind, uplifting.

Uses: Insect repellent, Excessive perspiration, Oily skin, Cold, flu, Minor infections, Fatigue, Headache, Migraine, Neuralgia, Tired feet, Rheumatic aches and pains, Softens skin.

Clary Sage

Note - Top to Middle

Type - Herb

Family - Labiatae

Part - Herb / Flowering tops and leaves

Extraction - Distillation

Aroma: Heavy herby and nutty.

Blends well With: Angelica, Basil, Bay, Bergamot, Cardamon, Cedarwood, Citronella, Coriander, Cypress, Frankincense, Geranium, Grapefruit, Jasmine, Juniper, Lavender, Lemon, Lime, Myrtle, Petitgrain, Rose, Sandalwood, Ylang Ylang.

Contraindications: Not before driving or operating heavy machinery, Not with Alcohol consumption, Large doses can cause headaches, Pregnancy, Epilepsy

Properties: Anticonvulsive, Antidepressant, Antiphlogistic, Antiseptic, Antispasmodic, Antisudorific, Aphrodisiac, Balsamic, Carminative, Deodorant, Digestive, Emmenagogue, Hypotensive, Nervine, Parturient, Sedative, Stomachic, Tonic, Uterine, hormone balancing, Kidney tonic, Soothing, Uplifting, Balance, Encourages hair growth, Astringent, Anti-inflammatory, Antibacterial, Powerful muscle relaxant.

Uses: Nervous tension, Anxiety, Uterine problems, Scanty periods, PMT, Menstrual cramps, Stress, Fertility, Digestive problems, Flatulence, Gastric spams, Headaches, Migraine, Tension, cramp, Excessive perspiration, TB, Asthma, Sore throats, Throat infections, Brings vigour after illness, Convalescence, Overcoming drug addictions, Depression and hopelessness, Cell regenerate, Scalp problems, Dandruff, Oily hair, Inflamed and puffy skin, Hypertension, Colds, Menstrual problems, Dry skin, Digestive problems.

Clove

Note -Base

Type - Spice

Family - Myrtaceae

Part - (Tree) Bud or Leaf

Extraction - Distillation

Aroma: Spicy, strong.

Blends well With: Basil, Benzoin, Black pepper, Cinnamon, Citronella, Grapefruit, Lemon, Nutmeg, Orange, Peppermint, Rosemary.

Contraindications: (Highly irritant), Sensitive skin, Pregnancy, Not for use with children

Properties: Analgesic, Anaesthetic, Antidontalgic, Antiemetic, Antineuralgic, Antiseptic, Antispasmodic, Aperitif, Aphrodisiac, Carminative, Caustic, Cicatrisant, Disinfectant, Insecticide, Parturient, Splenetic, Stimulant, Stomachic, Uterine, Vermifuge, Expectorant, Antihistamine, Aids digestion, Antidepressant, Parasiticide, Tonic for the Kidneys; spleen and stomach, Antibacterial.

Uses: Dyspepsia, Gum infections, Toothache, Bronchitis, Catarrh, Scabies, Athletes foot, Cold, Flu, Tinea, Acne, Bruises, Burns, Cuts, Ulcers, Wounds, Arthritis, Rheumatism, Sprains, Asthma, Colic, Nausea, Minor infection, Diarrhoea, Flatulence, General weakness, Muscular aches and pains, Tension, Scar tissue, Memory, Lethargy, Vomiting, Intestinal spasm, Halitosis, Headache, Respiratory problems, TB, Impotence, Frigidity, Helps child birth pains, Lupus.

Cypress

Note - Middle to base

Type - Wood

Family - Cupressaceae

Part - (Tree) Leaves and cones

Extraction - Distillation

Aroma: Woody and spicy, but refreshing and clear

Blends well With: Benzoin, Bergamot, Clary Sage, Juniper, Lavender, Lemon, Linden, Orange, Pine, Rosemary, Sandalwood.

Contraindications: High Blood pressure, Pregnancy,

Properties: Antiseptic, Astringent, Aids healing, Insecticide, Vaso-constricting, Tonic for circulatory system and liver, Cicatrisant.

Uses: Urinary problems, Fluid retention, Excessive perspiration, Diarrhoea, Menorrhagia, Tired aching legs, Oily skin, Rheumatism, Back ache, Haemorrhage, Swelling, Nasal congestion, Cold, Flu, Scars, Wounds, Haemorrhoids, Varicose veins, Asthma, Cellulitis, Menstrual cramp, Poor circulation, Spasmodic coughs, Dysmenorrhoea, Stress, Nervous tension, Acne, Eczema, Gum disorders, Incontinence, Menopausal problems, Nose bleeds, Whooping cough.

Eucalyptus

Note - Top

Type - Wood

Family - Eucalyptus globulus

Part - (Tree) leaves

Extraction - Distillation

Aroma: Clear, sharp and piercing

Blends well With: Benzoin, Cajeput, Cedarwood, Coriander, Cypress, Juniper, Lavender, Lemon, Lemongrass, Marjoram, Melissa, Peppermint, Pine, Rosemary, Star Anise, Teatree, Thyme.

Contraindications: Sensitive skin, Kidney problems, Toxic if taken internally, Heart problems, Not for children, High Blood pressure, Pregnancy, Epilepsy, Do not use if you are on any Homoeopathic medication.

Properties: Analgesic, Antirheumatic, Antipholgistic, Antiseptic, Antispasmodic, Antiviral, Antibacterial, Balsamic, Cicatrisant, Decongestant, Deodorant, Depurative, Diuretic, Expectorant, Febrifuge, Hypoglycemiant, Insecticide, Rubefacient, Stimulant, Vermifuge, Vulnerary, Parasiticide, Cools and soothes, Strengthens nervous system,

Uses: Respiratory complaints, Croup, Bronchitis, Ringworm, Insect bites, Shingles, Chicken pox, Herpes, Muscle aches and pains, Dysentery, Hay fever, Burns, Throat infections, Colds, Chest infections, Acne, Asthma, Boils, Cold sores, Cuts,

Fever, Flu, Lice, Laryngitis, Rheumatism, Skin infections, Sore throat, Urinary infections, Aids concentration, Catarrh, TB, Sinusitis, Migraine, Typhoid, Diphtheria, Malaria, Cystitis, Diarrhoea, Gall stones, Nephritis, Gonorrhoea, Diabetes, Haemorrhage, Neuralgia, Pyorrhoea.

Fennel

Note - Top to middle

Type - Herb

Family - Umbelliferae

Part - (Herb) seed

Extraction - Distillation

Aroma: Floral, herbal and spicy

Blends well With: Basil, Geranium, Lavender, Lemon, Rose, Rosemary, Sandalwood.

Contraindications : Pregnancy, Epilepsy, Toxic if used in large doses, not for babies.

Properties : Antiphlogistic, Antiseptic, Antispasmodic, Aperitif, Carminative, Detoxicant, Diuretic, Emmenagogue, Expectorant, Galactagogue, Insecticide, Laxative, Resolvent, Splenetic, Stimulant, Stomachic, Sudorific, Tonic, Vermifuge, Reduces lactobacillus, Has an action similar to Oestrogen, Stimulates lactation, Reduces the toxic effect of alcohol, Body cleansing and detoxifying.

Uses : Kidney Stones, Menstrual problems, PMT, Respiratory problems, Urinary tract infections, Flatulence, colic, Menopausal problems, Diuretic, Gout, Liver problems, Children's complaints, Intestinal parasites, Nausea, Vomiting, Indigestion, Cellulitis, Obesity, Odema, Rheumatism, Asthma, Bronchitis, Anorexia, Bruises, Dull skin, Oily skin, Alcohol poisoning, Appetite reduction, Arthritis, Colitis, Constipation, Fluid retention, Mouth and gum problems, Hangovers, Stomach ailments, Eases digestion, Hiccups, Whooping cough, Scanty periods.

Frankincense

Note - Middle to base

Type - Resin

Family - Burseraceae

Part - (Tree) Bark

Extraction - Distillation

Aroma: Woody, spicy, and a hint of lemon

Blends well With: Basil, Black Pepper, Cedarwood, Cinnamon, Citrus oils, Galbanum, Geranium, Ginger, Grapefruit, Lavender, Orange, Melissa, Myrrh, Neroli, Patchouli, Pine, Sandalwood, Vetiver.

Contraindications: Pregnancy.

Properties: Uterine tonic, Astringent, Blood coagulant, Calming, Deepens breathing, Induces sweating, Pulmonary antiseptic, Calming, Clears the lungs, Anti-inflammatory.

Uses: Bronchitis, Laryngitis, Asthma, anxiety, Stress, Emotional upsets, Urinary tract infections, Cystitis, Uterine tonic, Wounds, Mature skin, Blemishes, Dry skin, Scars, Catarrh, Dysmenorrhoea, Cold, Flu, Nervous tension, Acne, Coughs, Laryngitis, Meditation, Menstrual problems, PMS, Menorrhagia, Respiratory conditions, Scar tissue, Improves skin tone, genito-urinary infections, Catarrh, Nephritis, Genital infections, Uterine haemorrhage, Post natal depression, Calms during labour, Breast inflammation, Dyspepsia, Belching, Wrinkles, Oily skin, Ulcers, Carbuncles.

Geranium

Note - Middle

Type - Floral

Family - Geraniacea

Part - (plant) Flowers and leaves

Extraction - Distillation

Aroma: Sweet and heavy, a little like rose with a hint of mint.

Blends well With: Angelica, Basil, Bay, Bergamot, Carrot Seed, Cedarwood, Citronella, Clary Sage, Grapefruit, Hyssop, Jasmine, Lavender, Lemon, Lime, Mandarin, Marjoram, Neroli, Orange, Patchouli, Petitgrain, Rose, Rosemary, Sandalwood, Tea Tree.

Contraindications: Sensitive skin, Pregnancy.

Properties: Analgesic, Anticoagulant, Antidepressant, Aphrodisiac, Antiseptic, Anti-fungal, Anti-inflammatory, Astringent, Cicatrisant, Cytophylactic, Diuretic, Deodorant, Haemostatic, Hypoglycemiant, Insecticide, Styptic, Tonic, Vasoconstrictor, Vulnerary, Cleanses the body of toxins, Stimulates lymphatic system, Clears digestive mucous, Balances Sebum, Skin cleanser, Improves flow of blood.

Uses: Anxiety, Depression, Balances mind, Stress, PMT, Menorrhagia, Lack of vaginal secretions, Inflammation, Breast Congestion, Congested system, Jaundice, Kidney stones, Gallstones, Diabetes, Urinary infections, Fluid retention, Swollen ankles, Throat infections, Mouth Infections, Neuralgia, Gastritis, Colitis, Insect Repellent, Eczema, Shingles, Herpes, Ringworm, Chilblains, Oily skin, Sluggish skin, Congested skin, Cuts, Menopausal conditions, Cellulitis, Mastitis, Emotional problems, tonsillitis, Burns, Muscular aches and pains, Respiratory conditions, Rheumatism, Swelling, Ulcers, Apathy, Acne, Bruises, Broken capillaries, Dermatitis, Haemorrhoids, Lice, Mature skin, Mosquito repellent, Wounds, Engorgement of breasts, Poor circulation, Sore Throat, Nervous tension, Abscesses, Boils, Bronchitis, Indigestion, Insect bites.

Jasmine

Note - Middle to Base

Type - Floral

Family - Jasminacaea

Part - Flowers

Extraction - Enfleurage / Solvent Extraction

Aroma: Sweet and flowery.

Blends well With: Bergamot, Citrus oils, Chamomile, Clary Sage, Coriander, Frankincense, Geranium, Guaiacwood, Immortelle, Lavender, Mandarin, Melissa, Mimosa, Myrtle, Neroli, Orange, Palmarosa, Patchouli, Peppermint, Petitgrain, Rose, Rose wood, Sandalwood, Vetiver, Ylang Ylang.

Contraindications: Sensitive skin, Pregnancy, Not for Babies, Excessive use can cause problems with bodily fluids such as phlegm, May have a narcotic effect and cause lack of concentration.

Properties: Menstrual regulator, Sedative, Antidepressant, Stimulates lactation, Boosts confidence, Analgesic, Balances hormones, Increases male fertility.

Uses: Stress, Skin Care, Throat infections, Coughs, Catarrh, Listlessness, Apathy, Melancholy, Hopelessness, Menstrual cramps, Back pain, Labour Pain, Impotence, Frigidity, Dry Skin, Itchy skin, Muscle aches and pains, Child Birth, Lethargy, Nervous tension, PMS, Post natal depression, Vaginal infections, Premature ejaculation, Hoarseness.

Juniper

Note - Middle

Type - Herb

Family - Cupressacea

Part - Berries

Extraction - Distillation

Aroma: Slightly woody

Blends well With: Benzoin, Bergamot, Cedarwood, Citrus oils, Cypress, Frankincense, Geranium, Ginger, Grapefruit, Orange, Lavender, Lemongrass, Lime, Melissa, Pine, Rosemary, Sandalwood, Vetiver.

Contraindications: Pregnancy, Kidney problems, not for use with babies.

Properties: Antiseptic, Anti-rheumatic, Antispasmodic, Aphrodisiac, Astringent, Carminative, Cicatrisant, Clears Mucous from intestines, Depurative, Detoxicant, Digestive aid, Disinfectant, Diuretic, Emmenagogue, Nervine, Insecticide, Parturient, Regulating appetite, Regulating periods, Rubefacient, Stimulating, Stomachic, Sudorific, Tonic, Vulnerary.

Uses: Genito-Urinary infections, Cystitis, Strangury (Inability to pass urine), Kidney stones, Cellulitis, Dropsy, Fluid retention, releasing toxins, Piles, Obesity, Cirrhosis, Arthritis, Rheumatism, Gout, Sciatica, Stiff joints, Menstrual cramps, Childbirth, Problem skin, Oily skin, Congested skin, Seborrhoea, Acne, Blocked pores, Dermatitis, Eczema, Psoriasis, Swelling, Haemorrhoids, Ulcers, Stress, Oily Hair, Indigestion, Insomnia, Menstrual problems, Loss of appetite, Muscular aches and pains, PMS, Intestinal parasites, Colds, Flu, Anxiety, Purifying the blood, Circulation problems, Cough, Diarrhoea, Fatigue,

Lavender

Note - Middle

Type - Flower

Family - Labiatae

Part - Flowers

Extraction - Distillation

Aroma: Floral and slightly woody

Blends well With: Basil, Bay, Bergamot, Cedarwood, Chamomile, Citronella, Clary Sage, Cypress, Eucalyptus, Geranium, Grapefruit, Hyssop, Jasmine, Lemon, Lemongrass, Lime, Mandarin, Marjoram, Myrtle, Neroli, Nutmeg, Orange, Patchouli, Peppermint, Petitgrain, Pine, Thyme, Rosemary, Tea Tree.

Contraindications: Low Blood pressure, Early Pregnancy.

Properties: Analgesic, Anticonvulsive, Antidepressant, Antiphlogistic, Antirheumatic, Antiseptic, Antispasmodic, Antiviral, Bactericide, Balances central nervous system, Carminative, Cholagogue, Cicatrisant, Cordial, Cytophylactic, Decongestant, Deodorant, Detoxicant, Diuretic, Emmenagogue, Fungicide, Hypotensive, Increases gastric secretions, Nervine, Promotes growth of new skin cells, Restorative, Sedative, Splenetic, Stimulates bile production, Sudorific, Vulnerary.

Uses: Anger, Exhaustion, High blood pressure, Heart palpitations, Insomnia, Muscular spasm, Sprains, Strains, Rheumatic pains, Bronchitis, Asthma, Catarrh, Colds, Laryngitis, Throat infections, TB, Infections, Period pain, Scanty periods, Leucorrhoea, Childbirth, Cleanse spleen and liver, Nausea, Vomiting, Colic, Flatulence, Insect repellent, Burns, Sunburn, Acne, Eczema, Psoriasis, Abscesses, Boils, Carbuncles,

Fungal growths, Swelling, Scars, Gangrene, Alopecia, Headaches, Lice, fleas, Appetite stimulating, Whooping cough, Flu, Nervous Tension, Stress, Vertigo, Shock, Athlete's foot, Genito-urinary problems, Cystitis, Scalds, Wounds, Sores, Varicose veins, PMT, Ulcers, Spider bites, Ringworm.

Lemon

Note - Top

Type - Citrus

Family - Rutaceae

Part - Peel

Extraction - Expression / Distillation

Aroma: Citrus, Sharp and fresh

Blends well With: Bay, Benzoin, Black pepper, Cardamon, Chamomile, Citronella, Citrus oils, Eucalyptus, Fennel, Frankincense, Geranium, Ginger, Jasmine, Juniper, Lavender, Linden, Neroli, Peppermint, Rose, Sandalwood, Ylang-Ylang.

Contraindications: Sensitive skin, Phototoxic, High Blood pressure.

Properties: Antacid, Antisclerotic, Antiscorbutic, Antineuralgic, Antirheumatic, Antipruritic, Antiseptic, Astringent, Bactericide, Carminative, Cicatrisant, Decongestant, Depurative, Diuretic, Emollient, Escharotic, Febrifuge, Haemostatic, Hepatic, Hypoglycemiant, Hypotensive, Insecticide, Laxative, Stomachic, Tonic, Vermifuge.

Uses: Varicose veins, Easing blood flow, High Blood pressure, Anaemia, Restoring vitality to Red blood cells, Stimulating white corpuscles, Infectious diseases, Nosebleeds, Sore throat, Coughs, Colds, Flu, Fever, Cold sores, Herpes, Digestive complaints, Counteracting acidity in stomach, Diabetes, Cleanses body, Constipation, Cellulite, Headaches, Migraine, Neuralgia, Rheumatism, Arthritis, Insect bites and stings, Removes dead skin cells, broken capillaries, Cleansing greasy skin, Corns, Warts, Verrucae, Scars, Strengthens nails, Cuts, Circulation problems, Boosts immune system, Asthma, Bronchitis, Catarrh, Dyspepsia, Sinusitis, Tonsillitis, Chilblains, Mouth sores, Middle ear infections, Depression, Indigestion,

Boils, Debility, Fluid retention, Mouth Ulcers, Oily skin, Wounds.

Lemongrass

Note - Top

Type - Citrus

Family - Graminaea

Part - Leaves

Extraction - Distillation

Aroma: Strong, sweet and lemony

Blends well With: Basil, Cedarwood, Coriander, Eucalyptus, Geranium, Jasmine, Lavender, Neroli, Niaouli, Palmarosa, Peppermint, Rosemary, Tea Tree, Thyme, Vetiver, Yarrow.

Contraindications: Sensitive skin, use in low dose, High Blood pressure.

Properties: Antidepressant, Antiseptic, Bactericide, Carminative, Deodorant, Digestive, Diuretic, Fungicide, Galactagogue, Insecticide, Prophylactic, Stimulant, Tonic, Tones the skin, Sedative, Relaxing.

Uses: Exhaustion, Boosting parasympathetic nerves, Digestive complaints, Illness, Loss of appetite, Colitis, Indigestion, Gastro-enteritis, Infectious disease, Respiratory infections, Sore throat, Laryngitis, Fever, Aching muscles, Muscular aches and pains, Tired legs, Jet Lag, Headaches, Fatigue, Insect repellent, Fleas, Aids flow of breast milk, Open pores, Acne, Oily skin, Athlete's foot, Thrush, Digestive disturbances, Stress, Anxiety, Fluid retention, Gastric infections, Gout, Lice, Mental fatigue, Poor Circulation, Rheumatism, Scabies.

Lime

Note - Top

Type - Citrus

Family - Rutaceae

Part - Peel

Extraction - Expression / Distillation

Aroma: Sharp and Tangy

Blends well With: Angelica, Basil, Bergamot, Citronella, Citrus oils, Clary Sage, Geranium, Linden Blossom, Lavender, Neroli, Nutmeg, Palmarosa, Rose, Rosemary, Violet, Ylang Ylang.

Contraindications: Phototoxic, Sensitive skin.

Properties: Antiscorbic, Antiseptic, Antiviral, Apertif, Astringent, Bactericide, Disinfectant, Febrifuge, Haemostatic, Insecticide, Restorative, Tonic, Stimulating, Activating, Refreshing, Uplifting, Digestive stimulant, Stimulates appetite, Stimulates digestive secretions.

Uses: Apathy, Anxiety, Depression, Fever, Colds, Sore Throat, Flu, Coughs, Chest congestion, Catarrh, Sinusitis, Immune system tonic, Infections, Anorexia, Alcoholism, Rheumatic pain, Greasy skin, Acne, Cuts, Wounds, Anaemia, Brittle nails, Boils, Chilblains, Corns, Herpes, Insect bites, Mouth Ulcers, Spots, Varicose veins, Warts, Arthritis, Cellulitis, High Blood Pressure, Nose bleeds, Obesity, Poor circulation, Rheumatism, Asthma, Throat infections, Bronchitis, Dyspepsia, Headaches, Stress.

Mandarin

Note - Top to Middle

Type - Citrus

Family - Rutacaea

Part - Peel

Extraction - Expression

Aroma: Sweet and tangy

Blends well With: Basil, Bergamot, Black Pepper, Chamomile, Cinnamon, Citrus oils, Clary Sage, Coriander, Cumin, Geranium, Grapefruit, Juniper, Lavender, Lemon, Lime, Marjoram, Nutmeg, Palmarosa, Petitgrain, Rose.

Contraindications: Phototoxic.

Properties: Antispasmodic, Cholagogue, Cytophylactic, Digestive tonic, Emollient, Sedative, Tonic, Uplifting, Stimulates appetite, Stimulates liver, Regulate Metabolic processes, Aids secretion of Bile, Aids breaking down of fats, Calms the Intestines, Revitalising, Skin tonic.

Uses: Depression, Anxiety, Flatulence, Morning sickness, PMT, Stretch Marks and scarring, Digestive weakness, Good for children/pregnant women and the elderly, Insomnia, Nervousness, Acne, Oily skin, Fluid retention, Obesity, Hiccups, Restlessness, Constipation, Digestive problems.

Marjoram

Note - Middle

Type - Herb

Family - Labiatae

Part - Leaves

Extraction - Distillation

Aroma: Slightly Spicy

Blends well With: Basil, Bergamot, Cedarwood, Chamomile, Cypress, Eucalyptus, Geranium, Lavender, Mandarin, Melissa, Orange, Nutmeg, Peppermint, Rosemary, Rose wood, Tea Tree, Thyme, Ylang Ylang.

Contraindications: May cause drowsiness with prolonged use, Pregnancy.

Properties: Analgesic, Anaphrodisiac, Antiseptic, Antispasmodic, Carminative, Cephalic, Cordial, Digestive, Emmenagogue, Expectorant, Hypotensive, Laxative, Nervine, Restorative, Sedative, Tonic, Vulnerary, Calming, Dilates the arteries and capillaries, Cleanses toxins, Regulates Menstrual cycle, Hypnotic,

Uses: Stress, Anxiety, Psychological trauma, Confronting "issues", Grief, Loneliness, Hyperactivity, Muscular aches and pains, Lower back pain, Rheumatic aches and pains, Swollen joints, Stiff joints, After-sports rub, High Blood pressure, Headache, Migraine, Insomnia, Digestive problems, Stomach cramps, Indigestion, Constipation, Flatulence, Sea Sickness, Chest infections, Colds, Sinusitis, Bronchitis, Asthma, Congestion, Painful periods, Bruises, Sprains, Arthritis, Menstrual problems, Coughs, Colic, Chilblains, Ticks, Lumbago,

Strains, Dyspepsia, Leucorrhoea, PMS, Nervous tension, Cramps, Emotional comfort, Flu, Circulation.

Orange

Note - Top

Type - Citrus

Family - Citrus Vulgaris / Aurantium / Sinesis

Part - Peel

Extraction - Expression

Aroma: Zesty and refreshing citrus

Blends well With: Angelica, Black Pepper, Cedarwood, Cinnamon, Citrus oils, Coriander, Clary Sage, Clove, Cumin, Cypress, Frankincense, Geranium, Ginger, Hyssop, Jasmine, Juniper, Lavender, Myrrh, Neroli, Nutmeg, Petitgrain, Rose, Rose wood.

Contraindications: Sensitive skin, Phototoxic.

Properties: Antidepressant, Antiseptic, Antispasmodic, Carminative, Digestive, Febrifuge, Sedative, Stomachic, Tonic, Stimulates bile, Helps digestion of fats, Stimulates Appetite, Aids digestion of Vitamin C, Aids formation of collagen, Lowers cholesterol, Uplifting, Calming.

Uses: Depression, Tension, Stress, Boredom, Lethargy, "Butterflies" in the stomach, Diarrhoea, Constipation, Viral infections, Colds, Bronchitis, Fever, Repairing body tissues, Sore muscles, Rickety bones, Insomnia, Anxiety, Congested skin, Wrinkles, Dermatitis, Skin complaints, Flu, Oily skin, Coughs, Heartburn, Indigestion, Dull complexion, Dyspepsia, Mouth ulcers, Obesity, Palpitations, Water retention, Nervous tension.

Patchouli

Note - Base

Type - Herb

Family - Pogostemon patchouli

Part - Leaves

Extraction - Distillation

Aroma: Earthy and woody, a bit spicy (sort of mouldy)

Blends well With: Angelica, Bergamot, Black pepper, Cedarwood, Clary Sage, Elemi, Frankincense, Galbanum, Geranium, Ginger, Lavender, Lemongrass, Myrrh, Neroli, Orange Pine, Rose, Rose wood, Sandalwood, Ylang Ylang.

Contraindications: Sedative in low doses but Stimulating in high doses, May cause loss of appetite, May cause a headache in some people.

Properties: Grounding, Balancing, Antidepressant, Antipholgistic, Antiseptic, Anti-inflammatory, Aphrodisiac, Astringent, Cicatrisant, Cytophylactic, Deodorant, Diuretic, Febrifuge, Fungicide, Insecticide, Sedative, Tonic, Soothing, Calming, Opens pores, Cell regeneration.

Uses: Lethargy, Clarifying problems, Loose skin, Weight loss, Diarrhoea, Water Retention, Cellulite, Sweating, Insect bites and stings, Snake bites, Scars, Cracked skin, Sores, Wounds, Acne, Eczema, Fungal infections, Scalp disorders, Skin disorders, Athlete's foot, Dry Skin, Oily Skin, Tinea, Excessive Menstrual flow, Dandruff, Dermatitis, Hair care, Impetigo, Wrinkles, Frigidity, Nervous exhaustion, Stress, Anxiety, Bed sores, Depression.

Peppermint

Note - Top

Type - Herb

Family - Labiatae

Part - Leaves and flowering tops

Extraction - Distillation

Aroma: Minty

Blends well With: Basil, Benzoin, Cedarwood, Cypress, Eucalyptus, Jasmine, Lavender, Lemon, lemongrass, Mandarin, Marjoram, Niaouli, Pine, Rosemary.

Contraindications: (Very cooling on the skin - so best used in very small concentration on the skin), Sensitive skin, Pregnancy, Nursing Mothers (can discourage flow of milk), Should not be used with Homoeopathic remedies.

Properties: Analgesic, Antidontalgic, Anaesthetic, Antigalactagogue, Antiphlogistic, Antiseptic, Antispasmodic,

Astringent, Carminative, Cephalic, Cholagogue, Cordial, Decongestant, Emmenagogue, Expectorant, Febrifuge, Hepatic, Nervine, Stimulant, Stomachic, Sudorific, Vasoconstrictor, Vermifuge, Encourages sweating, Insecticide, Softens skin, Improves thinking, Uplifting.

Uses: Anger, Hysteria, Nervous trembling, Mental fatigue, Depression, Colds, Mucous, Fever, Respiratory disorders, Dry coughs, Sinus congestion, Asthma, Bronchitis, Cholera, Pneumonia, Tuberculosis, Food poisoning, Vomiting, Diarrhoea, Constipation, Flatulence, Halitosis, Colic, Gall stones, Nausea, Travel sickness, Kidney disorders, Liver disorders, Numbness in the limbs, Shock, Vertigo, Anaemia, Dizziness, Fainting, Headaches, Migraines, Toothache, Aching feet, Rheumatism, Neuralgia, Muscular aches, Scanty menstruation, Painful periods, Mastitis, Dermatitis, Ringworm, Scabies, Pruritus, Itching, Inflammation, Sunburn, Blackheads, Oily hair and skin, Abdominal cramps, Digestive upsets, Flu, Morning Sickness, Shingles, Insect bites, Nervous stress, Indigestion, Acne, Palpitations.

Rosemary

Note - Middle

Type - Herb

Family - Labiatae

Part - Flowering tops and leaves

Extraction - Distillation

Aroma: A strong refreshing herbal scent

Blends well With: Basil, Black Pepper, Cedarwood, Frankincense, Geranium, Ginger, Grapefruit, Hyssop, Lavender, Lemongrass, Lime, Mandarin, Melissa, Myrtle, Orange, Peppermint, Petitgrain, Pine, Tea Tree, Tangerine.

Contraindications: Pregnancy, High Blood pressure, Epilepsy, Not to be taken with Homoeopathic remedies.

Properties: Analgesic, Antidepressant, Antirheumatic, Antiseptic, Antispasmodic, Astringent, Carminative, Cephalic, Cholagogue, Cicatrisant, Cordial, Decongestant, Digestive, Diuretic, Emmenagogue, Hepatic, Hypertensive, Nervine,

Resolvent, Stimulant, Stomachic, Sudorific, Tonic, Vulnerary, Invigorating, Strengthens the mind, May help restore speech; hearing and sight, Heart tonic, Cardiac stimulant, Encourages hair growth.

Uses: Memory, Mental Strain, Dullness, Lethargy, Weakness, Mental exhaustion, Headaches, Migraines, Gastric problems, Vertigo, Paralysed limbs, Gout, Rheumatic pains, Tired and overworked muscles, Low blood pressure, Anaemia, Colds, Asthma, Chronic bronchitis, Flu, Hepatitis, Cirrhosis, Gallstones, Jaundice, Blocked bile ducts, Colitis, Dyspepsia, Flatulence, Stomach pains, Menstrual cramps, Scanty periods, Water retention, Cellulite, Obesity, Sagging skin, Skin congestion, Puffy skin, Swelling, Scalp disorders, Dandruff, Infections, Halitosis, Stress, Eyesight, Apathy, Muscle fatigue, Poor circulation, Aches and pains, Acne, Dermatitis, Eczema, Oily hair, Insect repellent, Lice, Seborrhoea, Scabies, Varicose veins, Rheumatism, Whooping cough.

Sandalwood

Note - Base

Type - Wood

Family - Santalaceae

Part - Inner wood

Extraction - Distillation

Aroma: Woody and Exotic

Blends well With: Basil, Benzoin, Bergamot, Black Pepper, Cedarwood, Cypress, Frankincense, Geranium, Jasmine, Lavender, Lemon, Mimosa, Myrrh, Neroli, Palmarosa, Patchouli, Rose, Rose wood, Vetiver, Ylang Ylang.

Contraindications: Depression? (May cause mood to drop lower, may act as an antidepressant)

Properties: Antiphlogistic, Antiseptic, Anti-inflammatory, Antispasmodic, Aphrodisiac, Astringent, Bechic, Carminative, Diuretic, Emollient, Expectorant, Sedative, Tonic, brings peace and acceptance, Stimulates immune system.

Uses: Nervous tension, Anxiety, Obsessional attitudes, Cutting ties with the past, Meditation, Genito-urinary problems,

Cystitis, Frigidity, Impotence, Chest infections, Sore throat, Dry coughs, Bronchitis, Lung infections, Insomnia, Catarrh, Heartburn, Diarrhoea, Dry skin, Oily skin, Aging skin, Dehydrated skin, Itching, Acne, Boils, Infected wounds, Cracked skin, Chapped skin, Shaving rash, PMS, Upset stomach, Stress, Urinary tract infections, Laryngitis, Nausea, Depression, Eczema, Fatigue, Respiratory problems, Skin problems, Sunstroke, Venereal infections.

Tea Tree

Note - Top

Type - Wood

Family - Myrtaceae

Part - Leaf

Extraction - Distillation

Aroma: Pungent and Sterile

Blends well With: Black Pepper, Cinnamon, Clary Sage, Clove, Coriander, Cumin, Cypress, Eucalyptus, Geranium, Ginger, Lavender, Lemon, Mandarin, Marjoram, Nutmeg, Orange, Pine, Rosemary, Thyme.

Contraindications: Sensitive skin, Pregnancy

Properties: Antibiotic, Antipuritic, Antiseptic, Antiviral, Antibacterial, Balsamic, Cicatrisant, Cordial, Disinfectant, Expectorant, Fungicide, Insecticide, Stimulant, Sudorific, Boosts immune system.

Uses: Shock, Infectious diseases, Eliminating toxins, Flu, Colds, Cold sores, Catarrh, Glandular fever, Gingivitis, AIDS (not a cure, but may boost immune system to be of benefit), Post-operative shock, Convalescence, Vaginal thrush, Genital infections, Urinary tract infections, Cystitis, Genital and anal pruritus, Chickenpox, Itching, Rashes, Insect bites and stings, Ear infections, Tonsillitis, Enteritis, Intestinal parasites, Infected wounds, Boils, Carbuncles, Spots, Acne, Shingles, Burns, Sores, Sunburn, Ringworm, Warts, Tinea, Herpes, Athlete's foot, Dry scalp, Dandruff,. Bronchitis, Verrucae, Asthma, Hysteria, Abscesses, Calluses, Blisters, Respiratory problems.

4

Planting of Medical and Aromatic Plants

The use of plant-based products for disease prevention and treatment has become increasingly popular in many societies. The World Health Organization (WHO) has estimated that about 80% of the population in developing countries rely chiefly on traditional medicine for their health care needs, of which a major portion involves the use of plant extracts (Azizol and Jamaludin, 1995)

With growing interest in medicinal plants as a source of new pharmaceutical products and the increasing demand for herbal products in Malaysia, it is expected that the demand for raw materials will also increased. Since most of the medicinal plants resources are from natural resources and many plant species are now facing extinction, it is of necessary to domesticate and cultivate selected species from both forest and non-forest areas. The success of such domestication programme will assist in the conversation of plant genetic resources, avoid further depletion and meet the demand for raw materials from the herbal industries.

Medicinal and Aromatic Plants of Malaysia

In Malaysia, the biodiversity of plant resources offers some 12 500 species of flowering plants and 5000 species of cryptograms. About 2000 species are recognized for their medical properties and they are still being used among certain communities (Latin, 1994). Some of these plants that are used as traditional medicines are also used as common spices or food additives. Species which have been commonly used for herbal preparations.

The aromatic plants like pepper, turmeric, ginger, cinnamomum, lemon grass etc. are exclusively used in the house-hold sector as natural food flavouring. Some of the aromatic plants which have the potential to be used in industry. Lately, the demand for natural aromatic resources is increasing in the international essential oil market. Essential oils which are obtained from the bark, leaves, flowers and fruits are natural sources for fragrance, flavour, species and medicine.

Some Commonly Used Medicinal Plantsa

Species	*Local name*	*Common use(s)*
Eurycoma longifolia	Tongkat Ali	Health tonic
Labisia pumila	Kacip Fatimah	Post-partum preparation
Centella asiatica	Pegaga	Health tonic
Curcuma xanthorizza	Temu lawak	Jamu
Andrographis paniculata	Hempedu bumi/ akar cerita	Herbal tea
Zingiber zerumbit	Lempoyang	Jamu
Eugenia aromatica	Cengkih	Toothpaste
Mentha arvensis	Pudina	Toothpaste
Curcuma domistica	Kunyit	Cosmetic, food additive
Cassia alata	Gelenggang	Antiseptic
Smilax myosotiflora	Ubi jaga	Health tonic
Morinda citrifolia	Mengkudu	Health tonic, past-partum preparation
Leptospermum flavescens	China maki	Health tonic
Fibraurea odoratum	Pokok kapal terbang	antiseptic

*Burkill (1996); Perry and Metzer (1980)

Some commonly used aromatic plantsa

Species	*Local name*	*Common use(s)*
Piper nigrum	Lada hitam	Flavour
Cympogon nardus	Serai wangi	Cosmetics, insect repellant
Kaempferia galanga	Cekur	Spice

Contd...

Species	*Local name*	*Common use(s)*
Lawsonia inermis	Inai	Cosmetics
Melaleuca cajuputi	Gelam	Analgesic
Baeckea frutescens	Rempah gunung	Fragrance
Ocimum basilicum	Selasih	Cosmetics
Jasminium sambac	Melati	Fragrance
Michelia champaca	Cempaka	Cosmetics
Blumea balsamifera	Sembung	Health tonic, lotion
Cinnamomum zeylanicum	Kayu manis	Spice, fragrance
Cinnnamomum sintoc	Medang sintoc	cosmetics

* Burkill (1996); Perry and Metzer (1980)

Medicinal and Aromatic Plant Industries

Statistics have shown that between 1986 and 1996, the total import value of medicinal and aromatic plants increased from RM 141 million and RM 431 million, respectively. In terms of total export, there was are significant increase from RM 5.9 million to RM 63 million over the same period. The imports of medicinal and aromatic plantscome mainly China, India and Indonesia while exports are largely to Singapore, Phillipines, Australia and Hong Kong. Under the spice category, garlic is the important import item (RM 119.5 milllion in 1996), whereas the export of ginger declined from RM 2.4 million in 1992 to RM 0.6 million in 1996 (Ng and Azmi, 1997).

In industry, medicinal plants and their parts are used in the form of extracts with high and standardised contents of active constituents for the pharmaceutical and natural products industries. Many Malaysian plants which have been traditionally used to treat certain ailments are now being processed using modern technology for the production of functional foods and tonics. These include Allium sativum (garlic), Centella asiatica (pegaga), Eurycoma longifolia (tongkat ali), Labisia pumila (Kacip Fatimah) and Zingiber officinale (halia).

Aromatic plants and their parts are the sources of essential oils, resin, turpentine, flavours and fragrances which can be used in the preparation of traditional medicines as well as in industry. Some of the important essential oils used in medicine are mint oil (Mentha arvensis), peppermint oil (Mentha piperita), eucalyptus oil (Eucalyptus spp.), citranella oil (Cymbapogon nardus) and cinnamon leaf oil (Cinnamomum zeylanicum). As for the international market, keruing oil (Gurjun balsam) has recently been used as fixative in perfumes by manufacturers in Singapore. Agar wood or gaharu from the karas tree (Aquilaria spp.) is sold as oleoresin infiltrated fragrant wood. It was reported that the highest grade gaharu was valued at US$ 27 400 in Dubai (Ng and Azmi, 1997).

Many of our local plants are also rich in aromatic compounds that can be used commercially as flavour and fragrance agents in beverages, food products, confectionery, toothpaste, cosmetics and medicinal preparations. These plants include kunyit (Curcuma domestica), serai makan (Cymbopogon citratus), serai wangi (Cymbopogon nardus), pandan (Pandanus odorus) and keso (Polygonum minus). Given the tremendous diversity of aromatic plant species available in Malaysia and the continuous demand for flavour and fragrance by industries, the economic potential of commercial application of these species is very promising.

Planting of Medicinal Plant

In Malaysia, medicinal plants are generally collected from the wild, with limited cultivation being carried out. This has lead to serious depletion of certain species and put some in danger of extinction. Interest has grown in the cultivation of medicinal plants for herbal use. However, to ensure satisfactory, returns from planting medicinal plants, plant selection must be focused on species highly demanded by the industry. Planting will depend on land availability but the following planting conditions can be recommended.

i. Planting under forest conditions which include virgin forest, logged-over forest and plantation forest: in forest where its resources have been removed (logged over forest), enrichment planting with selected medicinal plants is suitable and beneficial. In plantation forest, planting can be carried out in conventional forest plantations where selected medicinal plants are planted under forest species such as teak, pine, acasia, sentang (Azadirachta exelsa) and kara (Aquilaria malaccensis).

ii. Integration with agricultural crops: other then planting under forest conditions, medicinal plants can also be integrated with other commercial crops such as rubber and oil palm. Such crops are able to provide shade and artificial forest environment to the medicinal species, and

iii. Under open condition: under this condition, medicinal species that have high tolerance to high light intensities such as serai wangi may be planted.

When the Malaysian government announced its intention to boost the herbal industry, the Perak state government allocated a land area of 250 ha in Sg. Klah, Sungkai, Perak for a project to cultivate traditional crops (herb, spices and ulam). A series of long and short term medicinal and aromatic plants, have been identified for planting.

In another similar project, Lembaga Kemajuan Kelantan Selatan (KESEDAR) was selected to lead a project on the mass production of medicinal plants of commercial importance. A total area of 60ha have been allocated in Gua Musang, Kelantan for this project.

Some Economically Important Aromatic Plants

Tongkat Ali (Eurycoma longifolia, Simaroubaceae)

Tongkat Ali is also known as tunjang bumi, pasak bumi and penawar pahit. It has long been used in traditional medicine, especially by the Malays and Orang Asli. The roots are boiled and used as an aphrodisiac and tonic for men; it is also used for treating malaria and fever. This crop grows well in deep sandy loams mixed with plenty of organic matter. The roots can be harvested at the age of at least five years.

Kacip Fatimah (Labisia Pumila, Myrsinaceae)

Kacip Fatimah is a small, slighty woody herbaceous plant, which can be found in forest throughout Malaysia from the sea level up to about 150m altitude. A decoction of the roots is used for post-partum treatment, gonorrhoea and rheumatism. This plant can be propagated through seed and vegetative cuttings and can be harvested at the age of 7-8 months.

Mengkudu (Morinda Citrifolia, Rubicieae)

Mengkudu is a small tree which can grow up to 6m tall with few spreading branches. It grows well on clay loam in full sunlight or in some shade. It flowers and fruits all year round and can be propagated by stem cutting or seeds. The roots are boiled and the resultant decoction drunk to encourage the onset of menstruation. The leaves are heated over a small fire and applied to the chest to relieve cough or to be abdomen for mothers after childbirth.

Kadok (Piper Sarmentosum, Piperaceae)

Piper sarmentosum, known as daun kaduk is very popular in Malaysia and is often mistaken for its cousin Piper betel leaf plant. A decoction of the boiled leaves has been known to be effective in treating coughs, flu, rheumatism, pleurisy and lumbago. The root is a remedy for toothache and may be made into a wash for fungoid dermatitis on the feet. The leaves are also reported to contain antioxidant property.

Serai Wangi (Cymbopogon nardus, Graminiae)

Serai Wangi is the perennial crop which grows well in sandy loam in full sun and establishes itself quickly into a bush. Infusion of the leaves is sometimes used in herbal bath for mothers to regain health after childbirth. The essential oil obtained from this herb is also used extensively in cosmetics.

Daun Kesom (Polygonum minus, Polygonaceae)

Daun Kesom is a bushy herb to 50cm tall which can be found growing in shallow ditches and wet places. It thrives on sandy loam in full sun and flowers upon maturity. It can be propagated from stem-cutting or seeds and is often planted for flavouring in cooking due to its strong aroma. Atrong docoction of the fresh herb is taken foe indigestion and as a remedy for stomach pains.

Akar Cerita (Andrographis paniculata, Acanthacea)

Akar Cerita is known for its incredibly bitter taste so much so it is also called 'hempedu bumi' or 'bile of the earth'. It prefers rich loamy soils with some shade. It flowers frequently and can be propagated from stem-cuttings or seeds. A decoction of the leaves is often taken orally to cure diabetes and to reduce high blood pressure. A leaf poultice is applied topically to relieve itchy skin and insect bites. This herb is also said to be useful as a liver tonic to help detoxify toxins in our body.

Pegaga (Centella asiatica, Apiaceae)

Pegaga, a popular 'ulam' (salad) is a creeping herb with a long stolen. It grows well in the open partially shaded habitats and is often planted in small scale for its medicinal properties. A decoction of pegaga have been used to treat skin diseases, hypertension and to improve blood circulation. The stolon with stems and roots may be used for cultivation. The plant can be propagated vegetatively using the stolon. It is ready for harvesting six months after planting whereby clumps of plants can be easily dug up using small spade. Pegaga is also a popular ingredient in cosmetic products.

Medicinal and Aromatic Plants

Traditionally, raw materials of most medicinal and aromatic plants have been sourced from natural forests. Continuous extraction from this source without concerted efforts on replacement through replanting has inevitably led to the depletion of these important raw materials.

One of the key determinant of the future development of the medicinal and aromatic plants industries in this country is the sustainable supply of the raw materials. For continuous and sustainable supply of the raw materials, some forms of planting are deemed necessary.

A major limitation in the widescale planting of potentially high economic value crops such as medicinal and aromatic plants is the issue of the land availability. Land for the planting of any crop, used to be available in abundance but is currently getting scarce. Futher more, because environmental consideration, clearing of forests for the purpose of crop cultivation is currently not encouraged. There is a tremendous pressure to conserve our forests. In addition, a lot of our natural forests have been gazetted as permanent forests.

Even in new plantings, with the good price of palm oil, the focus is more on the planting of this crop. In addition, monoculture planting of medicinal and aromatic plants, although of potentially high value, may involve some form of biological and economic risks. With this scenario, it is therefore imperative that alternative forms of planting of medicinal and aromatic plants, are sought and considered.

One option available is on agroforestry (Mahmud, 1997a), a combining agricultural crops such as oil palm with medicinal and aromatic plants (Mahmud, 1997b, c) on the same piece of land. Under the concept of maximum land utilization and the need for diversification and alleviating potential risks in planting, medicinal and aromatic plants providing added value to the land. In any agroforestry planting system to be adopted, due consideration should be given to minimizing possible competitive effects between the various component species and the provision of conducive environments for the proper establishment and growth of all component species.

In view of this, various factors (Mahmud, 1997a) have to be taken into consideration in considering the integration of medicinal and aromatic plants with oil palm and these include:

i. Growth habits of forest species in terms of growth rates, crown shape and size etc.

ii. Growth requirements for light, moisture, nutrients, space etc., of all component species.

iii. Duration of growth

iv. Topography, either flat, undulating or hilly terrain.

v. Planting direction in terms of maximizing light transmission and capture.

Taking the above factors into consideration, the following are some illustrations and interim proposals on the integration of selected medicinal and aromatic plants with oil palm in an agroforestry system of planting.

Integration of Tongkat Ali with Oil Palm

Tongkat Ali which is targeted for harvesting at 4 to 6 years after planting, has a monopodial growth habit with very limited branching. It can be possibly be integrated with oil palm without having to modify the existing planting system of oil palm. In view of its simple growth habit, the Tongkat Ali can be planted in a single row at a distance of three metres apart in the interrow spaces.

The planting can be done either in every palm rows or in alternate palms rows with the density of the Tongkat Ali in varying with the planting system. Since the Tongkat Ali may require initial shade in its early stages of establishment, the Tongkat Ali can be introduced at one, two or three years after the planting of oil palm with the expanding oil palm fronds providing the initial shade. The price of dried root of Tongkat Ali is between RM 30.00 - RM 40.00 per kg.

Integration of Kacip Fatimah or Serai Wangi with Oil Palm

Kacip Fatimah is a small slightly woody herbaceous plant which is harvested for its roots at he age of 7 - 8 months after germination. Serai Wangi belongs to the grass family which survives as clumps with the stems harvested at eight months after planting. Both these plants can be integrated with oil palm, utilising the abundant space in between the palms.

The Serai Wangi can be introduced at the same time as planting of the oil palm and the Kacip Fatimah, because of the need for initial shade, at 0.5, 1 or 2 years after oil palm planting. Because of the shorter growth duration, high density planting of Kacip Fatimah and Serai Wangi can be practised when these plants are interplanted with oil palm.

To avoid possible competition, the planting should be confined in the interrow spaces at spesific distances from the palm rows. Depending on when these crops are introduced, as much as 2 to 3 harvests of the Kacip Fatimah and Serai Wangi can be achieved with this form of planting. The price of the dried root of Kacip Fatimah and fresh leaves of Serai Wangi is RM 30.00- RM 50.00 per kg and RM 1.20, respectively.

Conclusion

It is obvious that with land resource getting limited, integrating medicinal and aromatic plants with a high value crop such as oil palm through suitable agroforestry systems of planting, appears to be a viable and attractive option which should be seriously considered by the planting community. Under current scenario of limited land availability and the need to increase productivity and income, maximizing land use through agroforestry systems of planting compared to the traditional monoculture planting, offers an alternative option for the planting of potentially high value crops such as the medicinal and aromatic plants.

With the adoption of existing advanced agricultural plantation technologies in agroforestry systems of planting and the planting properly implemented, establishment and planting success of the medicinal an aromatic plants under oil palm will be somewhat assured.

In addition, by raising the awareness of the herbal industry on the commercial importance of medicinal products using raw materials from our tropical forest, the economic potential of these medicinal and aromatic plants will be increased. This will subsequently contribute to the development of herbal industries as well as medicinal plants research in this country.

5

Organic Essential Oils

Organic essential oils are derived from plants that have been grown without the use of pesticides, on land that has been certified by an authorised regulatory agent such as ECOCERT or the Soil Association.

Today, many aromatherapists and nurses prefer to use organic essential oils in their clinical treatments because they believe they have more healing power and vitality than conventional essential oils. There is also the issue of pesticide residues to be considered too, since they have far-reaching effects for both the environment, and our bodies.

Every one of our Organic Essential Oils has been analytically tested for purity and certified under one of the following official regulatory agencies:

- The Soil Association
- Nature et Progres
- ECOCERT
- Qualite-France SA
- Agrobio

Quinessence organic essential oils bring you unrivalled value for money because in most instances we have purchase them directly from the farms where they are produced, thereby cutting out the middle-man. We then pass these savings along to you, and in many cases our organic essential oils are not a great deal more expensive than many of our conventionally produced essential oils.

Further to the organic essential oils we purchase from around the world, an increasing selection of our Certified

Organic essential oils are now distilled on-site from medicinal herbs and plants that have been grown for Quinessence on a 500 acre farm in the United Kingdom.

Whilst our preference is for organically produced essential oils, we do accept that it has yet to be proven scientifically they are any more effective than their conventionally produced counterparts. But even if it was proven there is no difference between them, we would still not change our view on this matter. There is much more to this subject than just efficacy.

By purchasing organic essential oils from growers who use traditional farming practices, we are all contributing towards a more sustainable ecological environment for the future. Surely this is a sensible and worthwhile investment for our forthcoming generations?

A large amount of agricultural land has already been lost due to soil erosion, and in many places the overuse of aggressive agrochemicals has destroyed the delicate balance between wildlife and its natural habitat.

Discover more about the sources of Quinessence organic pure essential oils and the importance of buying organic by browsing other pages under this category.

Organic Status

To be certified as organic in the United Kingdom, a farm must first register with the Soil Association and then enter a 3 year conversion period. After this 3 year period an inspection is made by the Soil Association to establish that all regulations have been strictly observed. Only then is the farmer allowed to legally claim the product 'certified organic'.

The Quinessence range of Certified Organic essential oils are required to meet the following strict criteria:

- All crops have been botanically authenticated
- No chemical fertilisers - only farmyard manure used
- No chemical insecticides or fungicides were used
- Weeds were controlled by hand weeding

The term 'Organic' is defined by Law, and within the European Union organic farming it is governed by the European

Council Regulation (EEC) No 2092/91 and means that farmers must abide by a strict set of rules. Organic status is only awarded to producers who have been inspected and shown to comply with all the necessary organic standards.

For almost 15 years we have been building close working relationships with growers, distillers and suppliers to ensure that our pure essential oils are produced by plants from a certified botanical species that were not subjected to the use of pesticides or herbicides. This philosophy is continuing to develop with an ever expanding number of producers who share our convictions with regards to organic agriculture and biodiversity.

And this is precisely why we develop close working relationships with those growers who use traditional farming practices - to promote a more sustainable ecological environment for the future. Nowhere is this more true than in the United Kingdom, where we have forged allegiances with a network of farmers who are all dedicated to growing high quality, organic medicinal plants for the production of essential oils.

Why Buy Organic?

Organic agriculture was developed as a safe and sustainable farming system, to produce healthy crops and livestock without causing damage to environment. The use of genetically modified organisms is prohibited, as is the use of artificial chemical fertilisers and pesticides on the land, since they are harmful to the environment.

Put simply, organic farming could perhaps be described as using methods of crop and animal husbandry that work in harmony with nature as opposed to dominating it. Using safer methods to develop healthy fertile soil and growing a mixture of crops, the farm remains biologically balanced. This in turn encourages a wide variety of beneficial insects and wildlife that will act as natural predators to crop pests and enrich the soil with micro-organisms.

Soil Erosion

Biodiversity is the living element of the natural world, and it is vital that we work in harmony with Nature to maintain its delicate balance. A great deal of agricultural land has already been lost due to soil erosion, and in many places the overuse of aggressive agrochemicals has destroyed the delicate balance between wildlife and its natural habitat. Top soil takes hundreds of years to develop and can not be replaced easily.

The amount of pesticides sprayed on our food and land in one year has reached an estimated 4.5 billion litres in the United Kingdom alone. Pesticides do not only kill pests, they can also kill beneficial insects and plants and have a direct influence on the balance of the ecosystem. Many pesticides, especially the organophosphate and organochlorine family, do not break down very easily, and can be absorbed into the food chain and eventually eaten by humans. Only 10-15% of applied pesticides reaches the target pests, with 85-90% drifting downwind for up to a mile or more.

Diversity in Nature

Organic agriculture helps to increase the level of biodiversity not only on the farm, but across the adjacent countryside. This is because it uses tried and tested traditional farming practices including varied crop rotation, mixed systems, permanent pasture, no agrochemicals, use of farmyard manure and good hedge management. Recent research has shown that this practice supports and nurtures the diversity of animals and plants in the countryside, providing them with food, refuge and a space to live and breed.

This is why we develop close working relationships with those growers who use traditional farming practices, in order to promote a more sustainable ecological environment for the future. Using traditional methods, the farm remains biologically balanced, encouraging a soil rich in bio-organisms whilst sustaining a wide variety of beneficial insects and wildlife that act as natural predators for crop pests.

By supporting our organic farmers we are able to help increase this level of biodiversity whilst also providing our customers with ecologically sound products. This will also provide arable farmers with a much needed alternative to non-food crops at a time when many farms are no longer able to compete with cheaper imports.

Sources and Origins of our Oils

Sourcing and purchasing organic and conventional essential oils from remote areas around the world is not a job for either a novice or the faint-hearted, because mistakes can be very, very costly for a company, in terms of both money and loss of reputation. Financial losses can be regained, but company reputations tarnished due to supplying poor quality oils are not so easily recovered.

So we work hard all year round to ensure we preserve the quality and continuity of supply that our customers have come to expect. Keeping the supply chain as short as possible, cutting out the middlemen and meeting the people who grow the crops are all steps we must take to maintain our high standards.

It takes many years of training and practice to learn about the variability in therapeutic properties and the organic chemistry between a given species of plant. When we are procuring our oils, our search is targeted for those with high levels of bioactivity and a fine fragrance. Many essential oils have been 'adjusted' to meet the requirements of the perfumery or flavours industries, and whilst that may be acceptable for their requirements, it is certainly not for ours.

Growing Conditions

True experts at sourcing these natural raw materials know precisely where the finest herbs and essential oils are produced, but it takes many years to acquire this expertise and to also build up relationships with the producers and distilleries. In reality, few companies manufacturing or supplying aromatherapy products today have been in business long enough to have gained such vital expertise.

The fertility of the soil the plant was grown in, the genetic differences in the plant, the variety, cultivation practices, the climate, post-harvest handling and level of expertise used in the process of extraction will all have a significant effect on the resulting fragrance and bioactivity of an essential oil. This is why the country of origin is so important when it comes to the quality of an oil, since the climatic and soil conditions greatly affect the oil producing cells within the plant.

Lavender oil (Lavandula angustifolia) from France is a very good example; if you have several bottles of lavender from different suppliers try comparing them with one another, and note the differences. They will undoubtedly differ in aroma, chemical composition and therapeutic activity, and this can be for a number of reasons. These variations can be due to the altitude the plant was grown at, whether it was extracted from a population or clonal variety, or if it was produced organically. But there can be other reasons for variability as well.

Deception and Adulteration

It is quite common for lavender oil claiming its country of origin as France to have actually originated in Bulgaria or Croatia. Or it could be a mixture of oils from all three locations. And just to be clear; there is nothing wrong with the lavender oils produced in these countries - oils of excellent quality are produced in both regions, but they each have a different chemistry, odour profile and therapeutic action to that of French lavender. And a different bulk purchasing price that is considerably less than that of French lavender oil too!

Of course variations in quality can be due to blatant adulteration with synthetic or isolated chemicals, and this accounts for quite a large amount of poor quality essential oils that find their way into aromatherapy. This is usually the case with oils that have been adjusted to meet the required profile of the perfumery industry.

But what is merely 'adjustment' or 'sophistication' for one industry can be adulteration to another. Interfering with the chemistry of an oil to meet an odour profile may suit the perfumer, but it does no favours to the aromatherapist. To obtain classic textbook results you must use pure essential oils as nature intended or they will not be as therapeutically effective.

There can be absolutely no compromises with quality, and at Quinessence we remain committed to only sourcing the very finest that nature has to offer, extracted from organically grown products from ecologically sustainable sources. Of course this is not at all an easy task, but during the past 20 years we have set our own standards of excellence from which we never vary.

In today's fast-buck world, few other companies seem prepared to invest the time and money required to reach such exacting standards.

To discover more about the origins of Quinessence essential oils, you may like to visit the pages below.

- Chamomile Roman oil - United Kingdom
- Lavender oil - France
- Neroli oil - Tunisia
- Rose Otto - Bulgaria
- Yuzu oil - Japan

Tunisian Neroli Essential Oil

Neroli essential oil is extracted from the fragrant blossoms of the bitter orange tree (Citrus aurantium sub.sp amara), and has a beautiful aroma that appeals to men and women alike. In common with rose and jasmine, neroli oil is almost a complete fragrance in itself and forms the heart of one of the worlds most enduring perfumes, 'Eau de Cologne'.

Although neroli oil is produced in many countries such as Algeria, Egypt, France, Haiti, Italy, Morocco and Spain, the oils produced in France and Tunisia have always been considered to be the very finest and still command the highest price. At Quinessence, our preference is for Tunisian neroli oil.

Unlike much of its French counterpart, Tunisian bitter orange trees are not subjected to agrochemicals, simply because they are just too expensive for the smaller farmers to afford. Surprisingly, much of the neroli essential oil exported from Tunisia is produced from the blossoms of trees grown by small growing cooperatives and families, rather than from large-scale cultivation farms.

Origins and Folklore

It is believed that C. aurantium originated in South-East Asia, later spreading to North-Eastern India, Burma and China, and eventually finding its way via Arab traders to Africa, Arabia and Syria. From these regions it was taken to the Mediterranean by the Moors, and by the end of the 12th century it was cultivated in Seville, Spain, thereby leading to the common name for bitter oranges.

It is not known precisely when or where the oil was first extracted by steam distillation, but legend has it that during the 17th century in Italy, Anne Marie de la Tremoille (Orsini), who was duchess of Bracciano and princess of Nerola, first introduced neroli oil as a fashionable fragrance to high society. She used it whilst bathing and also to perfume her stationary, scarves and most famously, her gloves.

The fragrance obviously caught on, because in 1709, the Italian perfumer J. M. Farina launched his blend of neroli, bergamot, lavender, lemon, petitgrain and rosemary onto an unsuspecting world, naming it 'Eau de Cologne'. The rest as they say, is history.

Fragrant Assets

The bitter orange tree is a small evergreen that typically reaches a height of 3 metres (10ft) in cultivation, but may attain up to 6 metres (20ft) when growing in the wild. It has a smooth brown trunk, stout branches and flexible green twigs with rather blunt thorns, and has a more erect stature and compact crown than that of the sweet orange tree (Citrus sinensis).

The green twigs contain a significant amount of essential oil, and these along with the broad, ovate, glossy and highly aromatic leaves are used to produce petitgrain oil. The golden-yellow sour fruits are round or oval with a thick, heavily pitted skin that yield bitter orange essential oil by cold expression. This is a truly fragrant tree!

Critical Timing

Throughout April and May in Tunisia, prolific clusters of attractive, highly scented blossoms consisting of 5 petals and 24 yellow stamens begin to appear on the tree. Further to the beautiful oil within, these flowers also produce tasty nectar which proves irresistible to honey bees. The oil content of the flowers increases as they develop and bloom.

The flowering buds are usually harvested by hand early in the morning just as they begin to open - but only on warm, sunny days, because damp or overcast weather can have an adverse effect on the fragrance of the oil. It is absolutely critical that the buds are collected at the correct stage of maturity, because if they are plucked too soon the yield of oil will be lower and the resulting oil will have an unwanted 'green' note in the fragrance.

Conversely, if the buds have opened too far when they are gathered much of the precious volatile oil will evaporate during the process of transportation to the stills. Getting the timing wrong either way will have a severe detrimental effect on both the fragrance and value of the distilled essential oil.

Preparation and Extraction

Before transportation to the distillery, the collected buds must be carefully 'winnowed' by hand to remove all traces of stray leaves, twigs or similar plant debris. Failure to remove this unwanted material will again result in a tainted fragrance of sub-standard quality, thereby be unable to command the high price normally associated with Tunisian neroli.

Isolation of the essential oil is achieved by low-pressure 'cool' water-steam distillation which yields a pale yellow oil with an exquisite, fresh, fruity-floral aroma. Up to 20% of the essential oil is dissolved into the water during the process of distillation, and this is recovered by solvent extraction resulting in what is known as 'orange flower water absolute'.

Since this material consists mainly of the water-soluble components of the oil, the aroma is not very representative of the flower, but nontheless is still put to good use in the perfumery industry. Solvent extraction of the flowers produces a dark orange/brown viscous absolute with the most beautiful rich, warm and floral fragrance that closely resembles that of the blossoms.

Perfect for Skin

Appealing in aroma to both men and women, neroli is one of nature's most effective antidepressant oils, which together with its balancing and sedative properties makes it perfect for treating all types of negative emotional conditions, states of anxiety, menopause, and insomnia. This action may also in part explain the oils reputation as an effective aphrodisiac. Most problem skin conditions respond extremely well to treatments incorporating neroli, but for best results mix it with a hypoallergenic carrier lotion or base cream rather than a carrier oil. Used as part of a regular skin care routine, neroli improves elasticity, stimulates new cell growth, reduces thread veins, softens wrinkles and scars, and smells absolutely divine. The perfect skin care oil!

Bulgarian Rose Otto

The origin of the cultivated rose is often quoted as the Gulf of Persia, which is now known as Iran. From the 10th to the 17th century the rose industry was developed and dominated by Persia, and particularly in Shiraz, the famous city of poets and oriental culture.

From here the rose industry spread into Arabia, Mesopotamia, Palestine, Asia Minor (Anatolia) Greece, India, North Africa, and due to the conquering Moors reached as far as Spain. According to legend, in the 13th century R. damascena was brought from Damascus to Southern France by the returning Crusaders, although some experts believe it may have actually been R. gallica instead.

Valley of the Roses

During the 16th century, Ottoman (Turkish) merchants imported R. damascena for cultivation throughout the Balkan countries, including a newly founded town in Bulgaria that would eventually become known as Kazanlik. Kazan is the Turkish word for "still", and Kazanlik literally means 'the place of stills'.

A nearby valley provided the perfect environment for growing roses, thereby establishing what would in later years become the finest rose oil producing region in the world. This area is now called the 'Valley of the Roses', and during 1878 cuttings from the improved stock were returned to Anatolia and planted in Isparta and Burdur, where current rose production still thrives.

Throughout the 19th century, the Bulgarian rose oil industry reigned supreme, almost monopolising the entire world supply of rose oil. This monopoly would not be broken until the industry was nationalised due to dramatic changes in the political and economical climate after World War 2, when production fell into a steady decline. Today, it is believed that Turkey holds the record as the largest producer of rose otto, and only the oil from this country matches the quality and fine fragrance to that of Bulgaria.

Climatic Conditions

In Bulgaria, the rose blossoms of Rosa damascena begin to bloom around the third week of May, and will continue for three or four weeks depending upon climatic conditions. The yield of oil can be dramatically affected by the prevailing weather conditions - for example during very hot and dry weather the harvest may last only two weeks and the yield of the oil is lowered due to loss by evaporation. Conversely, during mild and humid weather the harvest time can be extended whilst at the same time increasing the oil yield.

The harvesting season starts as soon as the flowers begin to open and continues until all the roses have been gathered. In Bulgaria and Turkey the blossoms are still collected by hand in the time-honoured way, and are nipped just below the calyx (the green, outer protective cover). Collection begins at sunrise when the oil yield is at its highest, and should be completed by 10.00 am whilst the dew is still on the flowers. The flowers are initially placed into baskets, and then transferred to sacks for transportation to the distilleries.

Time is of the Essence

Whilst the harvesters are picking the flowers, other workers carefully transfer the flowers from the baskets to the transportation sacks where they are weighed, and all the relevant details are recorded since harvesters are paid by the weight of flowers picked. Each sack weighs approximately 25 kilos when full and is loaded onto horse drawn carriages, the backs of donkeys or less commonly, trucks!

The harvest is then transported to the distillery as quickly as possible, since the picked flowers will begin to deteriorate immediately as precious volatile oil begins to evaporate due to the heat of the sun. This in turn of course will lower the yield of the crop and push up the price of production.

Extraction

In Bulgaria during the early 1900's, virtually all rose oil was distilled on-site using direct-fire stills operated by the farmers. A suitable site would be chosen adjacent to the field and near a stream and the apparatus would be set up. Although this sounds rather primitive, the yield produced from this type of amounts to 1 kilo of oil for every 2,500 to 3,000 kilos of roses. Amazingly, this is a considerably higher figure than can be achieved by modern industrial distillation techniques!

Modern stills are made of copper and are heated with an open wood fire from below. The roses can not be distilled in the usual way by directly injecting steam, because the petals compact to form a large mass that the steam can not penetrate. Therefore the distillation techniques have been refined in various ways to overcome this problem.

During distillation a large amount of oil is absorbed into the distillation water, and this is known as the 'First Water'. The rose oil must be recovered from this water to produce an acceptable yield, and this is achieved by skilfully re-distilling the water to separate the oil; a process known as cohobation.

The amount of oil produced directly from distillation is as low as only 20% or 25%, the majority being recovered from the distillate water by cohobation. This ratio does vary depending upon certain factors, but is usually in the region of 25% 'direct oil' and 75% 'water oil'. The 'Second Water' remaining after the process of cohobation is then sold as rose hydrosol (aka floral water) or recycled in the still for the next batch of flowers.

The total yield of oil will depend upon several conditions; climate, the time of the harvest, condition of the flowers and the method of distillation. During the middle of the harvest period the yield is higher than at the beginning, and mild weather will result in a further increase in the oil produced. On average, Rosa damascena will yield 1 kilo of oil per 4,000 kilos of flowers using modern distillation processes. Under very favourable conditions only 2,600 kilos of roses may be required to produce 1 kilo of oil, whereas under less favourable conditions up to 8,000 kilos of flowers may be required to produce the same amount of oil.

Aromatherapy Bases

An advanced range of hypoallergenic, unfragranced base products enriched with the therapeutic, beautifying and revitalising qualities of botanical extracts to provide a single, high performance aromatherapy treatment for your clients.

The Quinessence Aroma-botanicals Base Collection is an advanced aromatherapy delivery system, specially formulated to unite the benefits of your essential oils with the beautifying and revitalising qualities of our natural, botanically enriched bases. Your aroma - our botanicals.

Pure and natural botanicals of Aloe Vera, Comfrey, Ginseng, Goldenrod, Shea Butter and Seaweed are used extensively to nourish, tone and beautify skin. At the same time, these revolutionary bases work as a traditional carrier to deliver your essential oils in one easy to use, high-performance treatment.

As a practicing clinical aromatherapist myself, I truly appreciate that the products used in your clinic must produce outstanding results for your clients, whilst also being safe on delicate or sensitive skin. Therefore, when developing this range I insisted on using only natural, vegetal ingredients that have a long and proven record of safety and efficacy.

We purposely avoided the use of any modern controversial ingredients that can irritate sensitive skins. Although 'miracle' ingredients such as AHA's and fruit acids promise great results, most of them have not been in general use long enough to discover any problems caused by long-term use on the skin. Every one of the botanical ingredients in this range has been used safely and effectively for centuries, and has been scientifically proven to possess highly beneficial effects.

When these active botanicals are combined with effective vegetable oils such as Centella asiatica, Jojoba, Rosehip and Carrot, they offer a huge range of skincare benefits. Of course, without essential oils it would not be true aromatherapy skincare, so we have ensured that our bases will easily absorb the addition of your essential oils to guarantee truly outstanding results.

Product stability is a crucial factor that must be considered when choosing which supplier you will be entrusting your reputation with. Adding essential oils or vegetable oils to an aromatherapy base that has not been specifically designed for this purpose can result in the product eventually destabilising and breaking down. Over time, the oil and water will separate out resulting in an unusable product, an unhappy client and possibly your reputation damaged.

Aroma-Botanicals are guaranteed to accommodate the addition of your essential oils or vegetable oils without causing separation or disturbing the integrity of the product. Once blended, you can rest assured your aromatherapeutic treatments will remain both highly effective and stable. To ensure suitability for the most sensitive of skin types, these light textured, non-greasy products do not contain any animal extracts, lanolin or harsh chemical preservatives, and are of course fragrance-free, hypo-allergenic and non-comedogenic.

And finally, as a long standing BUAV (British Union for the Abolition of Vivisection) approved manufacturer, I can assure you that every single product in the Quinessence Aromatherapy Collection is manufactured without causing any suffering to animals.

Aromatherapy

Aromatherapy, commonly associated with complementary and alternative medicine (CAM), is the use of volatile liquid plant materials, known as essential oils (EOs), and other scented compounds from plants for the purpose of affecting a person's mood or health. Aromatherapy is a generic term that refers to any of the various traditions that make use of essential oils sometimes in combination with other alternative medical practices and spiritual beliefs. It has a particularly Western currency and persuasion. Medical treatment involving aromatic scents may exist outside of the West, but may or may not be intended by the term 'aromatherapy'.

History: Aromatherapy has roots in antiquity with the use of aromatic oils. However, as currently defined, aromatherapy involves the use of distilled plant volatiles, a twentieth century innovation. The word, aromatherapy, was first used in the 1920s by French chemist Rene Maurice Gattefosse, who devoted his life to researching the healing properties of essential oils after a lucky accident in his perfume laboratory. In the accident, he lit his arm on fire and thrust it into the nearest cold liquid, which happened to be a vat of lavender oil. Immediately he noticed surprising pain relief, and instead of requiring the extended healing process he had experienced during recovery from previous burns—which caused redness, heat, inflammation, blisters, and scarring—this burn healed remarkably quickly, with minimal discomfort and no scarring.

The main branches of aromatherapy include:

- Home aromatherapy (self treatment, perfume & cosmetic use)
- Clinical aromatherapy (as part of pharmacology and pharmacotherapy)
- Aromachology (the psychology of odors and their effects on the mind)

Materials: Some of the materials employed include:

- *Essential Oils:* Fragrant oils extracted from plants chiefly through distillation (*e.g.* eucalyptus oil) or expression (grapefruit oil). However, the term is also occasionally used to describe fragrant oils extracted from plant material by any solvent extraction.
- *Absolutes:* Fragrant oils extracted primarily from flowers or delicate plant tissues through solvent or supercritical fluid extraction (*e.g.* rose absolute). The term is also used to describe oils extracted from fragrant butters, concretes, and enfleurage pommades using ethanol.
- *Phytoncides:* Various volatile organic compounds from plants that kill microbes. Many terpene-based fragrant oils and sulfuric compounds from plants in the genus "Allium" are Phytoncides, though the latter are likely less commonly used in aromatherapy due to their disagreeable smells.

- *Herbal Distillates or Hydrosols:* The aqueous by-products of the distillation process (*e.g.* rose water). There are many herbs that are used to make herbal distillates and they have culinary uses, medicinal uses and skin care uses. Common herbal distillates are rose, lemon balm and chamomile.
- *Infusions:* Aqueous extracts of various plant material (*e.g.* infusion of chamomile)
- *Carrier Oils:* Typically oily plant base triacylglycerides that are used to dilute essential oils for use on the skin (*e.g.* sweet almond oil)

Theory: When aromatherapy is used for the treatment or prevention of disease, a precise knowledge of the bioactivity and synergy of the essential oils used, knowledge of the dosage and duration of application, as well as, naturally, a medical diagnosis, are required.

In the English-speaking world, practitioners tend to emphasize the use of oils in massage. In the UK, America and Australia, aromatherapy tends to be regarded as a complementary modality at best and a pseudoscience at worst.

On the continent, especially in France, where it originated, aromatherapy is incorporated into mainstream medicine. There, the use of the antiseptic, antiviral antifungal and antibacterial properties of oils in the control of infections is emphasized over the more "touchy feely" approaches familiar to English speakers. In France some essential oils are regulated as prescription drugs, and thus administered by a physician. French doctors use a technique called the aromatogram to guide their decision on which essential oil to use. First the doctor cultures a sample of infected tissue or secretion from the patient. Next the growing culture is divided among petri dishes supplied with agar. Each petri dish is inoculated with a different essential oil to determine which have the most activity against the target strain of microorganism. The antiseptic activity manifests as a pattern of inhibited growth.

In many countries essential oils are included in the national pharmacopeia, but up to the present moment aromatherapy as science has never been recognized as a valid branch of medicine in the United States, Russia, Germany, or Japan.

Essential oils, phytoncides and other natural VOCs work in different ways. At the scent level they activate the limbic system and emotional centres of the brain. When applied to the skin (commonly in form of "massage oils" *i.e.* 1-10% solutions of EO in carrier oil) they activate thermal receptors, and kill microbes and fungi. Internal application of essential oil preparations (mainly in pharmacological drugs; generally not recommended for home use apart from dilution - 1-5% in fats or mineral oils, or hydrosoles) may stimulate the immune system.

Choice and purchase: Oils with standarized content of components (marked FCC, for Food Chemical Codex) have to contain X amount of certain aroma chemicals that normally occur in the oil. But there is no law that the chemicals cannot be added in synthetic form in order to meet the criteria established by the FCC for that oil. For instance, lemongrass essential oil has to contain 75% aldehyde to meet the FCC profile for that oil, but that aldehyde can come from a chemical refinery instead of from lemongrass. To say that FCC oils are "food grade" then makes them seem natural when in fact they are not necessarily so.

Undiluted essential oils suitable for aromatherapy are termed therapeutic grade, but in countries where the industry is not regulated, therapeutic grade is based on industry consensus and is not a regulatory category. Some aromatherapists take advantage of this situation to make misleading claims about the origin and even content of the oils they use. Likewise, claims that an oil's purity is vetted by mass spectrometer or gas chromatography have limited value, since all such testing can do is show that various chemicals occur in the oil.

Many of the chemicals that occur naturally in essential oils are manufactured by the perfume industry and are used to adulterate essential oils because they are cheaper. There is no way to distinguish between these synthetic additives and the naturally occurring chemicals.

The best instrument for determining whether an essential oil is adulterated is an educated nose. Many people can distinguish between natural and synthetic scents, but it takes experience.

Price: Oils vary in price based on the amount of the harvest, the country of origin, the type of extraction used (steam distillation, CO_2 extract, enfleurage), and how desirable the oil is. Indian Sandalwood (Santalum album) is considered more desirable than Australian Sandalwood (Santalum spicatum), based upon the aroma, and is twice as costly, mainly because the species that yields Indian Sandalwood essential oils is endangered. Organic and wild harvested essential oils also tend to be more expensive.

Popular uses:

- Basil is used in perfumery for its clear, sweet and mildly spicy aroma. In aromatherapy, it is used for sharpening concentration, for its uplifting effect on depression, and to relieve headaches and migraines. Basil oil has many chemotypes and some are known to be emmenagogues and should be avoided during pregnancy.
- Bergamot is one of the most popular oils in perfumery. It is an excellent insect repellent and may be helpful for both the urinary tract and for the digestive tract. It is useful for skin conditions linked to stress, such as cold sores and chicken pox, especially when combined with eucalyptus oil. Bergamot is a flavoring agent in Earl Grey tea. But cold-pressed Bergamot oil contains bergaptene, a strong photosensitizer when applied to the skin, so only distilled or 'bergaptene-free' types can be topically used.
- Black pepper has a sharp and spicy aroma. Common uses include stimulating the circulation and for muscular aches and pains. Skin application is useful for bruises, since it stimulates the circulation.
- Citronella oil, obtained from a relative of lemongrass, is used as an insect repellant and in perfumery.
- Tea tree oil and many other essential oils have topical (external) antimicrobial (*i.e.* antibacterial, antifungal,

antiviral, or antiparasitic) activity and are used as antiseptics and disinfectants.

- Eucalyptus oil
- Sandalwood oil
- Thyme oil
- Clove oil is a topical analgesic, especially useful in dentistry. It is also used an antiseptic, antispasmodic, carminative, and antiemetic.
- Lavender oil is used as an antiseptic, to soothe minor cuts and burns, to calm and relax, and to soothe headaches and migraines.
- Yarrow oil is used to reduce joint inflammation and relieve cold and influenza symptoms.
- Jasmine, Rose, Sandalwood and Ylang-ylang oil are used as aphrodisiacs.

Criticism: The consensus of the position of medical professionals in the U.S.A. and England is that while pleasant scents can be relaxing, lowering stress and offering related effects, there is insufficient scientific proof of the effectiveness of aromatherapy. Scientific research on the cause and effect of aromatherapy is limited, although in-vitro testing has revealed some antibacterial and antiviral effects. Some benefits that have been linked to aromatherapy, such as relaxation and clarity of mind, are quite subjective and may arise from the placebo effect. Like many alternative therapies, few controlled, double-blind studies have been carried out-a common explanation is that there is little incentive to do so if the results of the studies are not patentable. Customers should be aware that aromatherapy may be unregulated, depending on the country. There are some treatments generally accepted in Western medicine to give a form of relief for the airways in case of cold or flu, such as mint and eucalyptus essential oils.

Skeptical literature suggests that aromatherapy is based on the anecdotal evidence of its benefits rather than proof that aromatherapy can cure diseases. Scientists and medical professionals acknowledge that aromatherapy has limited scientific support but argue that its claims go beyond the data or that the studies are neither adequately controlled nor peer reviewed. If there can be positive effects, there can also be negative ones if used incorrectly or in bad combinations, especially with traditional pharmacology. Most medical professionals are concerned that people with maladies curable by contemporary medicine will revert to certain holistic medicines, such as aromatherapy, homeopathy and Ayurvedic medicine, and receive no benefit while their health could have been maintained with scientifically proven medicine.

The term "aromatherapy" has been applied to such a wide range of products that almost anything which contains essential oils is likely to be called an "aromatherapy product", rendering the term somewhat meaningless in that context.

Some proponents of aromatherapy believe that the claimed effect of each type of oil is not caused by the chemicals in the oil interacting with the senses, but that the oil contains a distillation of the "life force" of the plant from which it is derived that will "balance the energies" of the body and promote healing or well-being by purging negative vibrations from the body's energy field. Arguing that there is no scientific evidence that healing can be achieved, and that the claimed "energies" even exist, many skeptics reject this form of aromatherapy as pseudoscience or even quackery. In addition, there are potential safety concerns.

Since essential oils are so potent, many can irritate the skin and can cause toxic reactions like liver damage and seizures unless diluted with a carrier oil such as sweet almond oil, olive oil, hazelnut oil, and rosehip seed oil. Phototoxic reactions may occur with certain citrus oils such as lemon or lime .

Essential Oil

An essential oil is any concentrated, hydrophobic liquid containing volatile aroma compounds from plants. They are also known as volatile or ethereal oils, or simply as the "oil of" the plant material from which they were extracted, such as oil of clove. The term essential indicates that the oil carries distinctive scent of the plant, not that it is an especially important or fundamental substance. Essential oils do not as a group need to have any specific chemical properties in common, beyond conveying characteristic fragrances. They are not to be confused with essential fatty acids.

Essential oils are generally extracted by distillation. Other processes include expression, or solvent extraction. They are used in perfumes and cosmetics, for flavoring food and drink, and for scenting incense and household cleaning products.

Various essential oils have been used medicinally at different periods in history. Medical applications proposed by those who sell medicinal oils vary from skin treatments to remedies for cancer, and are often based on historical use of these oils for these purposes. Such claims are now subject to regulation in most countries, and have grown correspondingly more vague, to stay within these regulations.

Interest in essential oils has revived in recent decades, with the popularity of aromatherapy, a branch of alternative medicine which claims that the specific aromas carried by essential oils have curative effects. Oils are volatilized or diluted in a carrier oil and used in massage, or burned as incense, for example.

Production

Distillation: Today, most common essential oils, such as lavender, peppermint, and eucalyptus, are distilled. Raw plant material, consisting of the flowers, leaves, wood, bark, roots, seeds, or peel, is put into an alembic (distillation apparatus) over water, As the water is heated the steam passes through the plant material, vaporizing the volatile compounds. The vapours flow through a coil where they condense back to liquid, which is then collected in the receiving vessel.

Most oils are distilled in a single process. One exception is Ylang-ylang (Cananga odorata), which takes 22 hours to complete through a fractional distillation.

The water recondensed from the distillation process is referred to as a hydrosol, hydrolat, herbal distillate or plant water essence, which may be sold as another fragrant product. Popular hydrosols are rose water, lavender water, lemon balm, clary sage and orange blossom water. The use of herbal distillates in cosmetics is increasing. Some plant hydrosols have unpleasant smells and are therefore not sold.

Expression: Most citrus peel oils are usually expressed mechanically, or cold-pressed. Due to the large quantities of oil in citrus peel and the relatively low cost to grow and harvest the raw materials, citrus-fruit oils are cheaper than most other essential oils. Lemon or sweet orange oils that are obtained as by-products of the commercial citrus industry are even cheaper.

Prior to the discovery of distillation, essential oils (EO) were extracted by pressing.

Solvent Extraction: Most flowers contain very little volatile oil to undergo expression and their chemical components are too delicate and easily denatured by the high heat used in steam distillation. Instead, a solvent such as hexane or supercritical carbon dioxide is used to extract the oils. Extracts from hexane and other hydrophobic solvent are called concretes, which is mixture of essential oil, waxes, resins, and other lipophilic (oil soluble) plant material.

Although highly fragrant, concretes contain large quantities of non-fragrant waxes and resins. As such another solvent, often ethyl alcohol, which only dissolves the fragrant low-molecular weight compounds, is used to extract the fragrant oil from the concrete. The alcohol is removed by a second distillation, leaving behind the absolute.

Supercritical carbon dioxide is used as a solvent in supercritical fluid extraction. This method has many benefits, including avoiding petrochemical residues in the product. It does not yield an absolute directly. The supercritical carbon dioxide will extract both the waxes and the essential oils that make up the concrete. Subsequent processing with liquid carbon dioxide, achieved in the same extractor by merely lowering the extraction temperature, will separate the waxes from the essential oils. This lower temperature process prevents the decomposition and denaturing of compounds and provides for a superior product. When the extraction is complete, the pressure is reduced to ambient and the carbon dioxide reverts back to a gas, leaving no residue. Although supercritical carbon dioxide is also used for making decaffeinated coffee, the actual process is different.

Production Quantities: Estimates of total production of essential oils are difficult to obtain. One estimate, compiled from data in 1989, 1990 and 1994 from various sources gives the following total production, in tonnes, of essential oils for which more than 1,000 tonnes were produced.

Oil	*Tonnes*
Sweet orange	12,000
Mentha arvensis	4,800
Peppermint	3,200
Cedarwood	2,600
Lemon	2,300
Eucalyptus globulus	2,070
Litsea cubeba	2,000
Clove (leaf)	2,000
Spearmint	1,300

Essential Oil Use in Aromatherapy

Aromatherapy is a form of alternative medicine, in which healing effects are ascribed to the aromatic compounds in essential oils and other plant extracts. Many common essential oils have medicinal properties that have been applied in folk medicine since ancient times and are still widely used today. For example, many essential oils have antiseptic properties, though some are stronger than others.. In addition, many are claimed to have an uplifting effect on the mind, though different essential oils have different properties. The claims are supported in some studies and unconfirmed in others.

Dilution: Essential oils are usually lipophilic (literally: "oil-loving") compounds that usually are not miscible with water. Instead, they can be diluted in solvents like pure 100% ethanol (alcohol), polyethylene glycol, or oils.

Raw Materials: Essential oils are derived from various parts of plants. Some, like orange oil, are derived from any of several parts of the plant.

Berries

- Allspice
- Juniper

Seeds

- Almond
- Anise
- Celery
- Cumin
- Nutmeg oil

Bark

- Cassia
- Cinnamon
- Sassafras

Wood

- Camphor
- Cedar
- Rosewood
- Sandalwood

Rhizome

- Ginger

Leaves

- Basil
- Bay leaf
- Cinnamon
- Common sage
- Eucalyptus
- Lemon grass
- Melaleuca
- Oregano
- Patchouli
- Peppermint
- Pine
- Rosemary

- Spearmint
- Tea tree
- Thyme
- Wintergreen

Resin

- Frankincense
- Myrrh

Flowers

- Chamomile
- Clary sage
- Clove
- Geranium
- Hyssop
- Jasmine
- Lavender
- Manuka
- Marjoram
- Orange
- Rose
- Ylang-ylang

Peel

- Bergamot
- Grapefruit
- Lemon
- Lime
- Orange
- Tangerine

Root

- Valerian

Rose Oil: The most well-known essential oil is probably rose oil, produced from the petals of Rosa damascena and Rosa centifolia. Steam-distilled rose oil is known as "rose otto" while the solvent extracted product is known as "rose absolute".

Dangers: Because of their concentrated nature, EO's generally should not be applied directly to the skin in their undiluted or "neat" form. Some can cause severe irritation or provoke an allergic reaction. Instead, essential oils should be blended with a vegetable carrier oil (also referred to as a base or "fixed" oil) before being applied.

Common carrier oils include olive, almond, hazelnut and grapeseed. Common ratio of essential oil disbursed in a carrier oil is 0.5-3% (most less than 10%) and depends on its purpose. Some EO's including many of the citrus peel oils, are photosensitizers, increasing the skin's reaction to sunlight and making it more likely to burn.

Industrial users of essential oils should consult the material safety data sheets (MSDS) to determine the hazards and handling requirements of particular oils.

Pesticide Residues

There is some concern about pesticide residues in EO's, particularly those used therapeutically. For this reason, many practitioners of aromatherapy choose to buy organically produced oils.

Ingestion: While some advocate the ingestion of essential oils for therapeutic purposes, this should never be done except under the supervision of a professional who is licensed to prescribe such treatment. Some very common EO's such as Eucalyptus are extremely toxic internally. Pharmacopoeia standards for medicinal oils should be heeded. EO's should always be kept out of the reach of children. Some oils can be toxic to some domestic animals, cats in particular. Owners must ensure that their pets do not come into contact with potentially harmful essential oils.

Smoke : The smoke from burning essential oils may contain potential carcinogens, such as polycyclic aromatic hydrocarbons (PAHs). Essential oils are naturally high in volatile organic compounds (VOCs). The internal use of essential oils should be fully avoided during pregnancy without consulting with a licensed professional, as some can be abortifacients in dose 0.5-10 ml.

Media: In 2006, the German movie Perfume: The Story of a Murderer was made on the subject of essential oils. The story takes place in France in the 1700's.

Extraction (fragrance)

Fragrance extraction refers to the extraction of aromatic compounds from raw materials, using methods such as distillation, solvent extraction, expression, or enfleurage. The results of the extracts are either essential oils, absolutes, concretes, or butters, depending on the amount of waxes in the extracted product.

To a certain extent, all of these techniques tend to distort the odour of the aromatic compounds obtained from the raw materials. Heat, chemical solvents, or exposure to oxygen in the extraction process denature the aromatic compounds, either changing their odour character or rendering them odourless.

Maceration/Solvent Extraction

Certain plant materials contain too little volatile oil to undergo expression, or their chemical components are too delicate and easily denatured by the high heat used in steam distillation. Instead, the oils are extracted using their solvent properties.

Organic Solvent Extraction

Organic solvent extraction is the most common and most economically important technique for extracting aromatics in the modern perfume industry. Raw materials are submerged and agitated in a solvent that can dissolve the desired aromatic compounds. Commonly used solvents for maceration/solvent extraction include hexane, and dimethyl ether.

In organic solvent extraction, aromatic compounds as well as other hydrophobic soluble substances such as wax and pigments are also obtained. The extract is subjected to vacuum processing, which removes the solvent for re-use. The process can lasts anywhere from hours to months. Fragrant compounds for woody and fibrous plant materials are often obtained in this matter as are all aromatics from animal sources. The technique can also be used to extract odorants that are too volatile for distillation or easily denatured by heat. The remaining waxy mass is known as a concrete, which is mixture of essential oil, waxes, resins, and other lipophilic (oil soluble) plant material, since these solvents effectively remove all hydrophobic compounds in the raw material. The solvent is then removed by a lower temperature distillation process and reclaimed for re-use.

Although highly fragrant, concretes are too viscous - even solid—at room temperature to be useful. This is due to the presence of high-molecular-weight, non-fragrant waxes and resins. Another solvent, often ethyl alcohol, which only dissolves the fragrant low-molecular weight compounds, must be used to extract the fragrant oil from the concrete. The alcohol is removed by a second distillation, leaving behind the absolute. These types of essential oils, from plants such as jasmine and rose, are called absolutes.

Due to the low temperatures in this process, the absolute may be more faithful to the original scent of the raw material, which is subjected to high heat during the distillation process.

Supercritical Fluid Extraction

Supercritical fluid extraction is a relatively new technique for extracting fragrant compounds from a raw material, which often employs Supercritical CO_2 as the extraction solvent. When carbon dioxide is put under high pressure at slightly above room temperature, a supercritical fluid forms (Under normal pressure CO_2 changes directly from a solid to a gas in a process known as sublimation.) Since CO_2 in a non-polar compound has low surface tension and wets easily, it can be used to extract the typically hydrophobic aromatics from the plant material. This process is identical to one of the techniques for making decaffeinated coffee.

Due to the low heat of process and the relatively unreactive solvent used in the extraction, the fragrant compounds derived often closely resemble the original odour of the raw material. Like solvent extraction, the CO_2 extraction takes place at a low temperature, extracts a wide range of compounds, and leaves the aromatics unaltered by heat, rendering an essence more faithful to the original. Since CO_2 is gas at normal atmospheric pressure, it also leaves no trace of itself in the final product, thus allowing one to get the absolute directly without having to deal with a concrete. It is a low-temperature process, and the solvents are easily removed.

In supercritical fluid extraction, high pressure carbon dioxide gas (up to 100 atm.) is used as a solvent.

Ethanol Extraction

Ethanol extraction is a type of solvent extraction used to extract fragrant compounds directly from dry raw materials, as well as the impure oils or concrete resulting from organic solvent extraction, expression, or enfluerage. Ethanol extracts from dry materials are called tinctures, while ethanol washes for purifying oils and concretes are called absolutes.

The impure substances or oils are mixed with ethanol, which is less hydrophobic [than the solutes?] and dissolves more of the oxydized aromatic constituents (alcohols, aldehydess, etc.), leaving behind the wax, fats, and other generally hydrophobic substances. The alcohol is evaporated under low-pressure, leaving behind absolute. The absolute may be further processed to remove any impurities that are still present from the solvent extraction.

Ethanol extraction is not used to extract fragrance from fresh plant materials; these contain large quantities of water, which would also be extracted into the ethanol.

Distillation: Distillation is a common technique for obtaining aromatic compounds from plants, such as orange blossoms and roses. The raw material is heated and the fragrant compounds are re-collected through condensation of the distilled vapour

Today, most common essential oils, such as lavender, peppermint, and eucalyptus, are distilled. Raw plant material, consisting of the flowers, leaves, wood, bark, roots, seeds, or peel, is put into an alembic (distillation apparatus) over water,

Steam Distillation: Steam from boiling water is passed through the raw material for 60-105 minutes, which drives out most of their volatile fragrant compounds. The condensate from distillation, which contain both water and the aromatics, is settled in a Florentine flask. This allows for the easy separation of the fragrant oils from the water. The water collected from the condensate, which retains some of the fragrant compounds and oils from the raw material. This fragrant water is called hydrosol and is sometimes sold for consumer and commercial use. This method is most commonly used for fresh plant materials such as flowers, leaves, and stems. Popular hydrosols are rose water, lavender water, and orange blossom water. Many plant hydrosols have unpleasant smells and are therefore not sold.

Most oils are distilled in a single process. One exception is Ylang-ylang (Cananga odorata), which takes 22 hours to complete distillation. It is fractionally distilled, producing several grades (Ylang-Ylang "extra", I, II, III and "complete," in which the distillation is run from start to finish with no interruption).

Dry/destructive Distillation: The raw materials are directly heated in a still without a carrier solvent such as water. Fragrant compounds that are released from the raw material by the high heat often undergo anhydrous pyrolysis, which results in the formation of different fragrant compounds, and thus different fragrant notes. This method is used to obtain fragrant compounds from fossil amber and fragrant woods where an intentional "burned" or "toasted" odour is desired.

Expression

Expression as a method of frangrance extraction where raw materials are pressed, squeezed or compressed and the oils are collected. In contemporary times, the only fragrant oils obtained using this method are the peels of fruits in the citrus family. This is due to the large quantity of oil is present in the peels of these fruits as to make this extraction method economically feasible. Citrus peel oils are expressed mechanically, or cold-pressed. Due to the large quantities of oil in citrus peel and the relatively low cost to grow and harvest the raw materials, citrus-fruit oils are cheaper than most other essential oils. Lemon or sweet orange oils that are obtained as by-products of the commercial citrus industry are among the cheapest citrus oils.

Expression was mainly used prior to the discovery of distillation, and this is still the case in cultures such as Egypt. Traditional Egyptian practice involves pressing the plant material, then burying it in unglazed ceramic vessels in the desert for a period of months to drive out water. The water has a smaller molecular size, so it diffuses through the ceramic vessels, while the larger essential oils do not. The lotus oil in Tutankhamen's tomb, which retained its scent after 3000 years sealed in alabaster vessels, was pressed in this manner.

Enfleurage

Enfleurage is a two-step process during which the odour of aromatic materials is absorbed into wax or fat, then extracted with alcohol. Extraction by enfleurage was commonly used when distillation was not possible because some fragrant compounds denature through high heat. This technique is not commonly used in modern industry, due to both its prohibitive cost and the existence of more efficient and effective extraction methods.

Carrot Seed Oil

Carrot seed oil is the essential oil extract of the seed from the carrot plant. The oil is steam distilled from the dried fruit. The odour is a dry-woody, earthy sweet smell, a yellow or amber-coloured to pale orange-brown liquid. Carrot seed oil can be found in different formulas dealing with skin conditions. The oil assists in removing toxins and water build up, giving the skin a fresher tone.

In Aromatherapy

The light yellow to amber coloured essential oil distilled from the seeds (mostly in France, Egypt, and India) differs from the orange carrot oil produced from the root of the common edible carrot. Carrot seed oil nonetheless offers the same familiar scent. Diuretic and hepatic, carrot seed operates as a kidney and liver cleanser, particularly indicated for jaundice and hepatitis. Its depurative (detoxifying) properties are likewise effective for treating arthritis and rheumatism. As a diuretic remedy for genito-urinary ailments, carrot seed is indicated for gout, cystitis, and calculi as well as edema.

Carrot seed stimulates lymphatic circulation and is otherwise carminative and vermifuge, and an emmenagogic menstrual regulator. Its relaxing qualities are helpful in the treatment of premenstual tension. It is also considered a blood tonic indicated for anemia.

As a dermal agent, carrot seed lends its depurative qualities to skin and body care preparations and procedures. A natural tanning agent and skin toner that protects aged and wrinkled skin, carrot seed is also remedial for dermatitis, eczema, psoriasis, and various rashes. It can be used topically to treat boils, abscesses, and skin ulcers.

Anethole

Anethole (or trans-anethole) is an aromatic compound that accounts for the distinctive "licorice" flavor of anise, fennel, and star anise. It may also be referred to as p-propenylanisole, anise camphor, isoestragole, or oil of aniseed. It is unrelated to glycyrrhizic acid, the compound which makes licorice taste sweet. The full chemical name is trans-1-methoxy-4-(prop-1-enyl)benzene. The chemical structure is shown at right. Chemically, it is an aromatic, unsaturated ether.

Anethole appears as white crystals at room temperature. Its melting point is 21 °C, and its boiling point is 234 °C. It has a chemical formula of C10H12O, and is closely related to estragole, an aromatic compound found in tarragon and basil. Anethole is distinctly sweet as well as having its flavoring properties and is measured to be 13 times sweeter than sugar. It is perceived as being pleasant to the taste even at higher concentrations.

It is slightly toxic and may act as an irritant in large quantities. It can stimulate hepatic regeneration in rats, and can also produce spasmolytic activity in high doses. It is a chemical precursor for paramethoxyamphetamine (PMA), which has been sold as ecstasy resulting in several deaths.

Eucalyptol

Eucalyptol is a natural organic compound which is a colourless liquid. It is a cyclic ether and a monoterpene. Eucalyptol is also known by a variety of synonyms: 1,8-cineol, limonene oxide, cajeputol, 1,8-epoxy-p-menthane, 1,8-oxido-p-menthane, eucalyptol, eucalyptole, 1,3,3-trimethyl-2-oxabicyclo[2,2,2]octane, cineol, cineole.

Composition: Eucalyptol comprises up to 90 percent of the essential oil of some species of eucalyptus (*e.g.* Eucalyptus polybractea), hence the common name of the compound. It is also found in bay leaves, mugwort, sweet basil, wormwood, rosemary, sage and other aromatic plant foliage. Eucalyptol with a purity from 99.6 to 99.8 percent can be obtained in large quantities by fractional distillation of eucalyptus oil.

Health Warning: In common with all volatile oils (essential oils), eucalyptus oil is toxic if ingested internally.

Properties: Eucalyptol has a fresh camphor-like smell and a spicy, cooling taste. It is insoluble in water, but miscible with ether, ethanol and chloroform. The boiling point is 176 °C and the flash point is 49 °C.

Uses: Because of its pleasant spicy aroma and taste, eucalyptol is used in flavourings, fragrances, and cosmetics. It is also an ingredient in many brands of mouthwash and cough suppressant.

Eucalyptol has been demonstrated to be capable of reducing inflammation and pain. It has also been found to be able to kill leukaemic cells.

Cineol was shown to be an effective treatment for Non-purulent sinusitis in a placebo controlled trial. Laryngoscope. 2004 Apr;114(4):738-42. PMID: 15064633 [PubMed - indexed for MEDLINE] 76 patients per treatment group were assigned to cineole or placebo. The dosage of the active ingredient was two 100-mg capsules of cineole three times daily. Symptom scores were significantly reduced in the cineole group. The mean values for the symptoms-sum-scores in the cineole group were 6.9 +/- 2.9 after 4 days and 3.0 +/- 2.8 after 7 days, and in the placebo group, 12.2 +/- 2.5 after 4 days and 9.2 +/- 3.0

after 7 days. Treated subjects experienced less headache on bending, frontal headache, sensitivity of pressure points of trigeminal nerve, impairment of general condition, nasal obstruction, and rhinological secretion. Side effects from treatment were minimal.

In a 1994 report released by five top cigarette companies, eucalyptol was listed as one of the 599 additives to cigarettes. It is added to improve the flavor.

Aromatherapy

Aromatherapy is the ancient science of healing, relaxing and energizing by the use of plants and their parts. The roots, barks, flowers, fruits, seeds and nuts play a crucial part in this science. It is one of the more popular branches of alternative medicines. The word aromatherapy is derived from two words aroma which means smell and therapy which stands for healing.

Essential oils form the basis of aromatherapy. These essentials oils are the extracts of plants and their parts and form their life force. These oils are extracted by the means of steam distillation, cold expression, or fixed oil or alcohol extraction. They are highly concentrated and should not be used directly. These oils can be blended together and this blend is called synergy. The synergy is more potent than the individual oils combined. To reduce the potency of these oils, you can dilute them by mixing them with carrier oils.

These oils affect your mood. They enter through our olfactory system and affect the nervous system, thus improving mood and relaxing or energizing us. This helps is alleviating stress and speeding up healing. These essential oils also have cosmetic properties and can be used in skincare and hair care products. Many of these oils have known anti-viral, antifungal and antiseptic properties. They are also used in household products for cleaning and antiseptic uses. These oils can be inhaled, massaged onto your body, added to the bath or shower or sprayed in the room.

The essential oils used in aromatherapy are the life force of the plants from which they have been extracted. These oils can be massaged on your body, inhaled, added to your bath or sprayed in the air. When you take "Aromatherapy massage" with the essential oils, these oils are absorbed into the bloodstream via the skin.

Aromatherapy Essential Oils

Aromatherapy oils are popularly known as essential oils. You can use these oils for health, beauty, relaxation and cooking. You can mix two or more essential oils together to form a synergy, while mixing two or more oils together to the vegetable oil can give you blend. You can get the water left after extraction of the oil called hydrosol and use it for healing and beauty purpose. Do not use essential oils directly. Always dilute them with the carrier oils before application. Use only the minimum recommended drops. These oils can be used for cooking and baking, in lieu of vegetable oils and also to add essence to your food. But you need to be careful since these oils are highly volatile. Always keep these oils away from the heat and electric sources as they are highly inflammable. Do not let the children and the pets touch these oils.

What are Essential Oils?

Aromatherapy oils are known as essential oils. These oils are the concentrated extracts of plants and their roots, stems, flowers and fruits. These oils form the base of aromatherapy and influence your body, mind and spirit. Any fragrance that uses an animal product like musk is not pure aromatherapy oil. Similarly, fragrances and perfumes too do not categorize as essential oils though they may smell similar to the aromatherapy oils and do not carry the therapeutic value.

Aromatherapy oils or essential oils are extracted from the plants usually by the means of distillation. The plant matter is treated with steam to soften the plant, break down its tissues and release the pure essential oils. The steam is then cooled down since it contains the essential oils and the water is separated from the oil. This oil is then filtered to get pure aromatherapy oil.

Sometimes they can also be extracted by pressing the part of the plant. *E.g.* if you twist the rind of a lemon or orange, you get a smelly liquid which is the essential oil of the fruit and can be extracted by the presses. The price of aromatherapy oils varies greatly, depending on the number of plant parts used in manufacture.

The greater the number of part plants used higher is the price. Also the oils extracted from the exotic plants are expensive. Lemon oil is cheaper since the rind of lemon contains a lot of oil. But the lavender oil is expensive because flowers contain very little oil and it takes about 45 kilograms of lavender flowers to extract a pound of lavender essential oil. Jasmine, rose and lavender are the most expensive of aromatherapy oils.

Only a few pure essential oils like lavender and tea tree can be applied directly to the skin. The rest of the oils are concentrated and must be diluted by mixing up with carrier oils which are made from nuts and seeds like apricot kernel, grape seed and jojoba, before application.

You can benefit from the use of aromatherapy oils in wide variety of ways like inhaling the oil, massaging it on your body and by soaking yourself in the bath water to which are added the essential oils. Massaging the oil onto the body is the most common method of getting the benefit of aromatherapy oils, since skin is the largest absorption organ that you have.

Oil Profiles

Aromatherapy makes use of different types of essential oils for curing different problems. Essential oils are extracted natural plants and herbs found the in nature. Discovered in the year 1930 by a French scientist it heals people using the aromas of different plants and herbs. Since essential oils are natural and herbal they are completely safe and do not have any negative side effects.

Angelica Root: Its botanical name is Angelica archangelica. It is extracted by steam distillation. Its colour is pale yellow and it's a thin liquid. It is mainly use for dull skin, exhaustion, gout, toxin buildup, water retention etc. It is phototoxic therefore should be avoided during pregnancy and diabetes.

Anise: Its Botanical Name is Pimpinella anisum. It is extracted by steam Distillation. Its colour is clear and it is a thin liquid. It is used for Bronchitis, colds, coughs, flatulence, flu, muscle aches, rheumatism. Those who have hypersensitive skin should avoid using it. It should also be avoided in endometriosis and estrogen-dependent cancers. It is narcotic and slows circulation if taken in large doses.

Basil: Its botanical name is Ocimum basilicum. It is extracted by steam Distillation. Its colour is clear and it is a thin liquid. It can be used for Bronchitis, colds, coughs, exhaustion, flatulence, flu, gout, insect bites, insect repellent, muscle aches, rheumatism, and sinusitis. High doses of basil may be carcinogenic due to its methyl chavicol content. It should be avoided during pregnancy and liver problems.

Cedarwood Atlas: Its botanical name is cedrus atlantica. It is extracted by steam Distillation. It is light golden yellow in colour and a medium oily liquid. It could be used for Acne, arthritis, bronchitis, coughing, cystitis, dandruff, dermatitis, stress. It should be avoided during pregnancy.

Eucalyptus: Its botanical name is eucalyptus globules. It is extracted by steam Distillation. Its colour is clear and it is a thin liquid. It could be used for Arthritis, bronchitis, catarhh, cold sores, colds, coughing, fever, flu, poor circulation, and sinusitis. It is very toxic when taken orally.

Uses for Essential Oils

Essential oils are the oils extracted from the natural plants and herbs. Aroma of these essential oils is used for aromatherapy. Discovered in the year 1930 by French scientist, aromatherapy is a very good natural technique for rejuvenating human mind and body. The aroma of essential oils directly affects the mental and physical health of the patient. Essential oils also help in creating emotional balance in emotionally disturbed people. These essential oils are highly volatile therefore one need to take great care for storing them.

Some of the essential oils are:

Eucalyptus, Sandalwood, Cedarwood, etc. All essential oils have different characteristics and hence are used for curing different types of disease. Essential oils could be used for curing physical and mental problems of people. It could be used for perfumes, room sprays, toners, shampoos, soaps etc. On the emotional front essential oils such as bergamot, chamomile, juniper, lemon, could be used for easing aggression. Oils such as Jasmine and Rose can be used to ease jealously. Essential oils such as marjoram and Benzoin are helpful for relaxing a person suffering loneliness. Essential oils such as cedarwood, ginger and fennel are effective in treating fear. Essential oils are effective in easing many other unpleasant emotions.

Essential oils can also be used for skin care and treating asthma, warts etc. Apart from curing and healing diseases, essential oils could be used for many other purposes. At home essential could also be used to fragrance wardrobe, book shelves.

It could also be used for preparing insect repellent. Add about 20 drops of essential oils to carrier oil like almond for massaging the body. To keep bookworms away from the books keep patchouli oil near the old books. Spicy oils added to a kettle or simmering water could be used to humidify and freshen the house.

How to Use Essential Oils

You can use aromatherapy essential oils at home or work place in a number of ways. Some of the common ways are:

> *Aroma therapy Inhalation - Is a process where you add 2-3 drops of essential oil into boiling water and inhale the steam, by covering your head with a towel to stop the steam from escaping. This also opens the pores of the skin and so more oil is absorbed giving the benefits of a facial.*

You can place the same bowl containing hot water and aroma oil under your bed so that your entire room is surrounded with aromatic fragrance. Handkerchiefs sprinkled with a drop or two of aroma oil is also beneficial. Similarly a tissue with aromatic oil can also be kept inside a pillow or cushion to have a relaxed and peaceful sleep.

Diffusers or Vaporizers: Diffusers are usually made of clay. They have an opening where you can place candles or earthen lamps. The top portion is like a cup useful for holding water and a few drops of aromatic oil.

Fill in the cup with water, few drops of aromatic oil. Then light candle or lamp filled with castor oil so that it burns for a longer time. The whole atmosphere is filled with fragrance once the water and oil heat up and evaporation takes place for nearly 6 hours. This can be used wherever scented air is required like gatherings, hotels, living rooms and even bedrooms. When the right essential oil is used there is an instant relief from pain and a relaxed positive feeling prevails.

Vaporizers are the insect repellents normally used in the forms of mats can be reused by the addition of 2-3 drops of essential oil and lighting them electrically. Slowly the soothing aroma is dispersed in the entire room. Citronella is used for repelling the insects lavender for bedroom, lemon or rosemary are useful for offices. Tea-tree due to its antiseptic property can be used to disinfect a sick room.

Massage : Aromatherapy Massage gives us the simultaneous double benefits of touch therapy with scent therapy. Massage tones the muscles, releases energy from tense muscles, detoxifies toxins and above all, improves blood circulation. There is a sense of pleasure and well being when you inhale the fragrance. During massage a high amount of oil is able to penetrate through the skin. Usually aroma oils are mixed with carrier oils like olive oil, sweet almond, sesame, coconut, sunflower and vegetable oil. Aroma oils should be used only after dilution, 10 drops or 1 tsp of essential oil can be mixed with 30ml of carrier oil for a rejuvenating effect.

Baths: You can add only a few drops of the selected aromatherapy bath oil to your bathtub or bucket. Stir well since some of the aroma oils are insoluble in water and spend 20 minutes in the tub. The aroma oil enters the body through the skin and gives a relaxed lasting effect.

Foot Bath: After a hard days work you can have a very refreshing feeling by dipping your feet in a bowl of lukewarm water with 2-3 drops of essential oil. This is useful even for sweaty and smelly feet.

Pot Pourri : This is a combination of dried flowers, herbs grass and seed pods to which a few drops of essential oil is added and kept in a bowl to give aromatic fragrance for 4-6 weeks. Another method is to keep the pot pourri mixture along with the essential oil in a container overnight and open the box the next morning so that the aroma spreads in the entire area.

Bed Time : 2-3 drops on the pillow cover while sleeping, is useful in treating headaches, stress, tension and in boosting confidence.

Essential and Organic Oils

Amrette Seed: These have warmth- giving, relaxing and stimulating properties. 2-3 drops of oil are used to relieve anxiety, depression, tiredness and other stress related conditions, cramps, pains and muscular aches. Can freshen up tired and hurting feet. Should be used in low dosage and frequent massages and bath with it should be avoided.

Aniseed: Have warming and stimulating properties. 3-5 drops are helpful in treating bronchitis, coughs and catarrh.

Angelica: Angelica is useful in muscular pains and aches, rheumatism, flu, cold, cough and aides digestion. Used in healing smoker's cough. Not to be used during pregnancy and avoid exposure to sunlight.

Basil: Have uplifting and refreshing properties. Has multiple uses 2-3 drops help to relieve tension, stress, mild anxiety, loss of appetite, indigestion, flatulence, nausea, temporarily relieves cough, sinusitis, cold, fever, bronchitis, earaches, eases rheumatic, arthritic, muscular pains and spasm. It also used as an insect repellent. But is to be avoided during pregnancy.

Bergamot: (3-5 drops) Has calming, refreshing and rejuvenating properties. Can heal wounds, relieves ulcers, treats pre menstrual tension and eczema. Acts as an appetizer. Relieves respiratory infections, colic, flatulence and indigestion. Used in oily skin problems. Used in treating mental and psychological disturbances. It is effective in treating cold sores and chicken pox. Acts as an antiseptic for urinary tract problem. Can be photosensitive and can cause skin irritation.

Black Pepper: Can be warming and strengthening. 2-3 drops can relieve stiffness, pains, muscular aches and fatigue.

Helps in curing heartburn, indigestion, flatulence, colic and loss of appetite. Tones muscles and helps in peripheral circulation. Increases concentration and alertness. Provides temporary relief from respiratory infections, chills, cold, flu, arthritis, fibrosis and catarrh. But should used in moderation.

Camphor: Should be used in moderation. Helps in treating colds, coughs, fever, constipation, arthritis, rheumatism, sprains, insomnia, acne, inflamed skin and depression. 2-3 drops can be used at a time.

Cardamom: 2-3 drops can be used. It is a tonic and helps to relieve aches, headaches, coughs, nausea and indigestion. But should be used in moderation.

Chamomile : (3-5) drops can give a soothing effect. Used for diarrhea, gastritis, colitis, urinary tract infection, menopause and menstrual related problems. Eases fear, anxiety and anger. It is helpful in treating sleeplessness and helps to relieve muscular and joint pains and is used in treating skin problems. Soothes inflamed wounds, broken capillaries, blisters. It can be used to lighten fair hair. Has mild effect on children facing teething problem and earache.

Clove Bud: 1-2 drops when used have warming and soothing properties. It is used as an effective antiseptic, analgesic and anti-bacterial. It provides relief from sprains, asthma, cold, flu, dyspepsia, diarrhea, toothache, ulcers, wounds, bronchitis, nervous tension, depression and stress. It is useful in fighting acne and acts as mosquito repellent. It should be used in low moderation and is to be avoided during pregnancy.

Cypress: 2 drops of this can provide refreshed, calm and strengthening effect. It brings down external bleeding, excessive perspiration and heavy menstrual flow; used as an astringent to circulation, hemorrhoids, varicose veins; useful in asthma, bronchitis, dry cough, cold and flu. Helps to heal swollen breasts. It should not be used during pregnancy.

Clarysage : Clarysage has Euphoric, sensual, warming and relaxing properties. 2-5 drops can be used. Brings down high blood pressure and excessive sebum. It is useful in dealing with anxiety, stress, tension and migraine, menstrual cramps and pain, PMT, muscular tension and excessive perspiration. It encourages labour and eases childbirth. Immune system is strengthened and reduces asthma. Causes drowsiness, so it has to be avoided if one suffers from epilepsy or in case of pregnancy.

Eucalyptus: 2-3 drops of this have cooling and clearing properties. It cures cold and fever. Clears blocked nose and head. Relieves stress, fatigue, muscular pains, sprains, aches, rheumatism, headaches, sinusitis and mild respiratory infections. It has anti-inflammatory and antibacterial properties too. And is also used as an insect repellent. Sometimes it can cause skin irritation.

Fennel have calming effect. 2-3 drops are useful in easing colic, constipation, nausea, flatulence, loss of appetite, fluid retention, menstrual pain, PMT, menopause and digestion problems. Has mild laxative and diuretic effect. Cures kidney stones and relieves intestinal spasm. Increases flow of breast milk, relieves bronchitis and helps to fight hangovers. It is to be avoided during pregnancy.

Frankincense it has strengthening and soothing properties. 3-5 drops can be used at a time. Helps in meditation. Strengthens emotionally against grief, fear and nightmares. It cures asthma, bronchitis, coughs and catarrh. It helps in healing dry, wrinkled, scarred, inflamed skin, ulcers and infected wounds. It helps to maintain supple skin.

Geranium : It is associated with calm, balancing, relaxing and refreshing properties. 5-7 drops helps to deal menopausal problems, postnatal depression, PMT. Normalizes skin imbalances and problems. Treats swollen and painful breasts, fluid retention problems, throat infections. It cures cold, flu, acne, bruises, burns, cuts, mouth ulcers, eczema and dermatitis. It acts as astringent and cleanser. Also works as insect repellent.

Ginger: 2-3 drops have warm and stimulating properties. Helps in blood circulation, aids memory, relaxes blood vessels. If inhaled, relieves morning sickness. Relieves pains, aches, sprains and strains. Cures cold, catarrh, flu, fever and sore throat. Relieves flatulence, travel sickness, indigestion. It may cause irritation in sensitive skin so use in moderation.

Juniper Berry: 2-3 drops can be used to heal bruises, acne, colic, cramps, menstrual pain, cough, arthritis, less menstrual flow, swollen and painful breasts. Tones the skin and deals with obesity, loss of appetite, hemorrhoids, poor circulation and fluid retention. If used in excess can irritate kidneys. Not be used if suffering from high B.P. and in pregnancy.

Lavender: It has harmonizing, soothing, balancing, refreshing, relaxing and calming properties. 5-10 drops relieves muscular aches and pains, bites and stings. Cures cold, flu, sleeplessness, headache and minor burns. It helps in relieving anxiety, stress and irritability. It helps to balance and harmonize the body. Usage should be avoided during pregnancy.

Lemon: 3-6 drops help in healing cold, fever, flu, sore throat, mouth ulcers, poor circulation, high B.P., hormonal headaches, wounds, stress, nervous tension, acidity and bronchial problems. Helps to stop hot flushes during menopause. Helps to clear freckles and is an effective insect repellent too. Avoid using it in sunlight.

Lemongrass: (1-3 drops) It helps to open the skin pores, treating oily skin, curing acne and indigestion. Helps in shock, grief and stress. Helps to fight lethargy, insomnia and irritability during menopause, excitability in children. Improves skin elasticity, scars and stretch marks. It gives relief from sore throat, headaches and mild respiratory problems. Can cause skin irritation. To be avoided during pregnancy.

Marjoram: (3-5 drops) Calming to the nervous system. Heals bruises and reduces sexual urges. Relieves anxiety, stress, high B.P., cold, flu, sinusitis, arthritis, rheumatism and swollen joints. Cures indigestion, constipation, flatulence, migraines, stomach and menstrual cramps. Use in limit and avoid during pregnancy.

Neroli: (1-3 drops) Helps in shocks, trauma, grief, stress, menopause and PMT. Cures dryness, improves elasticity of the skin. Calms restless children. Helps to lighten stretch marks and scars. Helps during pregnancy and labour.

Orange (sweet): (2-3 drops) Gentle on children and brings down fever. Eases constipation and diarrhea. Treats nervous tension, stress and anxiety, effective in healing mouth ulcers. Gives relief from bronchial coughs, colds, flu and insomnia. Avoid using under sunlight.

Palmarosa: (4-5 drops) Relieves cold, flu, indigestion, viruses and reduces fever. Helpful in treating acne, scars, dermatitis, maintains supple skin. Stimulates circulation, cell regeneration and appetite.

Peppermint: (1-3 drops) Cools skin inflammation, burns and sunburns. It is a decongestant and gives relief from cold, fever, flu, asthma, headaches, travel sickness, sinusitis, nausea, toothaches, stomach upsets, indigestion and hangover. Avoid during early pregnancy and on sensitive skin.

Patchouli: (2-4 drops) Helps to heal chapped rough skin, inflamed skin, wounds and sores. It is effective in treating dandruff and scars. Helps to relieve anxiety, stress and depression. Used in perfumery due to its exotic aroma. It is used as insect repellent. Excess dose should be avoided as it can cause sedation.

Petit grain: (4-5 drops) It builds resistance against illness. Helps in stimulating digestion and poor memory. Reduces excess acne and sweating, treats greasy hair and skin. It aids in reliving mental strain, anxiety, stress, flatulence, dyspepsia, restlessness and constipation.

Pine: (1-3 drops) It heals cuts and abrasions, excessive perspiration. Relieves colds, coughs, flu, sore throats, asthma, bronchitis, sinusitis, catarrh, muscular aches, arthritis, rheumatism, poor circulation, stress, fatigue, sciatica and poor concentration. Also used to repel insects.

Rose: (1-4 drops) Useful for dry, chapped, aging skin and eczema. Relieves asthma, dry cough, nausea, shock, poor circulation and palpitations. Used to treat irregular heavy menstruation, menstrual pain, PMT, irritability, impotence. Also helps in easing depression, tension, headache, frigidity and insomnia.

Rosemary: (2-4 drops) Improves concentration while studying. It clears dandruff and lice, adds luster to hair. Useful in relieving stress, anxiety, muscular aches and pains, rheumatism, arthritis, sinusitis, migraine, cold, flu, asthma, respiratory problem, poor circulation, menstrual cramps and scanty flow. Avoid usage if suffering from B.P. or epilepsy and during pregnancy.

Sandalwood: (2-5 drops) Heals dry, chapped, cracked, inflamed, mature, aging skin, acne, scars and blemishes. Acts as a deodorizer. Excites the senses. Helps to relieve dry coughs, sore throat, bronchitis, stress, depression, tension, anxiety, insomnia, and travel sickness. It is also an effective insect repellent.

Tarragon: (2-3 drops) It is anti-spasmodic, antiseptic and slightly diuretic. Useful in treating stomach disorders, indigestion, constipation, flatulence, cramps, PMT and nervousness.

Tea Tree: (2-5 drops) helpful in treating colds, flu, cold sores, shock, burns, bacterial and viral infections, nappy rash, stings, herpes, hysteria and in healing fungal and yeast infections.

Thyme (White) : (2 drops) A good stimulant and expectorant. Helpful in relieving cold, coughs, tension, anxiety, fatigue, skin irritation, headaches, rheumatic aches and pains. Also an useful insect repellent.

Vetiver: (1-3 drops) Heals cuts, wounds, blemishes and acne. Helpful in relieving stress, sprains, tension, muscular aches, pains, arthritis, rheumatism, stiffness, palpitations and congestion.

Ylang Ylang: (2-3 drops) Useful in skin care, high B.P., insomnia, PMT, menopause, impotence, frigidity, scalp conditioner. Helps to relieve stress, anxiety, tension, uncontrolled anger, rapid breathing and heart rate. If taken in excess it may cause headache and nausea. Not to be used before driving.

Essential Blends

Aromatherapy is one of the best natural therapies used to rejuvenate mind and body. It makes use essential oils - oils extracted from plants and herbs. It is a combination of two words "aroma" which means scent and "therapy" which means treatment. Aromatherapy was discovered by a French scientist in 1930.

The aroma of the essential oils directly affects the mental and physical health of the patient. Aromatherapy oil also helps in creating emotional balance in emotionally disturbed people. Some of the essential oils are eucalyptus, cedarwood, sandalwood, rosemary etc. Essential oils are highly volatile and therefore should be stored in an airtight container. Essential oils should be mixed with the career oil before using.

Every essential oil has its own unique application and is very effective when used for that purpose. How ever one could also blend 2 or more essential oils to get greater effect than those oils would give individually, when essential oils are blended in this way they are known as essential blends. Essential blends are the undiluted essential oils blended carefully to have a certain effect on mind and body. Essential oils must be blended cautiously. One must keep in mind for what purpose the oils are being blended.

For example, if one is blending oils for diabetes oils like angelica root should be avoided as they are not good for diabetes patient. For blending only natural products as such as essential oils, grain alcohol, carrier oils, herbs and water are used. Basically essential oils can be categorized in to 9 basic categories, Floral Woodsy, Earthy, Herbaceous, Minty, Spicy, Oriental and Citrus. Generally oils in the same category blend well together. Care must be taken that contradictory essential oils are not mixed to create an essential blend *e.g.* an energizing essential oil should not be blended with a relaxing essential oil.

Essential Organic Aromatherapy Oils

Synergies are the blends of organic aromatherapy oils. They are formed by mixing the various organic aromatherapy oils in different proportions or by mixing these oils with the right carrier oils. The power of each oil is magnified when blended together. These synergies can be added to your baths, inhaled, massaged or vaporized for getting the therapeutic benefits of the organic aromatherapy oils. These synergies have beautiful aromas and these smells combined with the soothing effects of the massages and baths produce the relaxation that you have wanted and thus promoting good health by the means of stress reduction.

- o *After Flight Synergy:* This synergy uses the blend of geranium, ginger and ylang ylang. Drop a few drops on your tissue or sprinkle them in your bath or shower to eliminate the after flight tiredness.
- o *Anti Pollen Synergy:* if you are allergic to the pollen, use the synergy of eucalyptus radiate, lemon and chamomile roman. You get the best results by inhaling the drops or using them in a vapouriser. If you are unable to do so, you can add these drops to your bath or mixed with a carrier oil for massage.
- o *Antiseptic Synergy*—You can get the antiseptic synergy by blending together the organic aromatherapy oils of tea tree, lavender and manuka. This is an excellent first aid kit.
- o *Anti-virus Synergy*—The combination of ravensara, tea tree and cedar Virginian has excellent anti-viral properties and hence are ideal for use during the colds and any other viral infections. This blend is warming, soothing and clearing to the nose and throat and can be used in bath, inhaled or vaporized.
- o *Breathe Easy Synergy*—A blend of cypress, pine and frankincense is refreshing and clearing for you after travelling through the polluted streets. Inhale a few drops on a tissue or vaporize it for immediate relief.
- o *Cellulite Synergy*—Tone the skin and increase circulation by blending juniper berry, sweet fennel and cypress. It helps the body break down the fatty deposits. Add a few drops to your bath or massage it on your skin.
- o *Energizing Synergy*—Blend grapefruit, pine and litsea cubeba to energize yourself after a tiring day. Recharge your batteries while driving by sprinkling a cotton ball with a few drops of this blend.
- o *Foot Ease Synergy*—Blend peppermint, benzoin and patchouli to revive your feet after a tiring day.

- *Head Ease Synergy*—Inhale or vapourize the blend of lavender, peppermint and chamomile roman to ease the head tensions.
- *Immune Optimize Synergy*—Geranium, tea tree and lemon when blended together give a powerful boost to your immune system. Add a small amount to your bath, vapourise it or add to a carrier oil for the massage.
- *Joint Mobility Synergy*—Keep your joins smooth and healthy by using a synergy of ginger, juniper berry and chamomile german. Add a few drops to the bath or to the carrier oil for massage.
- *Menopause Synergy*—Use the blend of geranium, clary sage and cypress for relief.
- *Muscle Ease Synergy*—The blend of marjoram sweet, rosemary and lavender when added to a carrier oil for massage or to the bath water will provide immediate relief to your tired, aching muscles.
- *Pre-menstrual Synergy*—If you suffer from pre-menstrual symptoms, use the blend of geranium, marjoram sweet and chamomile german. Add this blend to your bath or to a carrier oil for massaging your abdomen during these stressful feminine times.
- *Problem Skin Synergy*—Use the blend of lavender, bergamot and chamomile roman to cure red, dry, itchy skin. You can add this blend to any lotion before use.
- *Relaxing Synergy*—Soothe your nerves by using a blend of ylang ylang, chamomile roman and neroli which can be added to the bath.
- *Restful Sleep Synergy*—The blend of bergamot, clary sage and sandalwood when added to the bath will give you a peaceful sleep as this blend contains the most relaxing oils known in aromatherapy.
- *Sinus Synergy*—Keep your sinuses clear and healthy by using the blend of silver fir, eucalyptus radiate and basil. Inhale the drops from a tissue or use it in vaporizer.
- *Stress Synergy*—Use the blend of basil, juniper and geranium to soothe and relax the mind and body. Basil

is an excellent tonic for the mind to give it strength and clarity.

- o *Uplifting Synergy*—An elevating blend of grapefruit, bergamot and geranium will lift your spirits if you are depressed. It aids in concentration while driving.

Carrier Oils

Carrier oils are commonly known as base oils or vegetable oils. They are used to dilute the essential oils, CO2s and absolutes before being used on the skin or added to aromatherapy bath oils. These oils are called carrier oils because they carry the essential oils to the skin. The properties of different oils are different. You need to choose your carrier oil wisely to get the desired therapeutic effect.

These oils are generally cold-pressed vegetable oils. They are obtained from the fatty portions of the plant like nuts and seeds. While aromatherapy bath oils are highly volatile and fragrant, these carrier oils do not evaporate or release strong smells. Never use the commercially available vegetable oils in aromatherapy.

This is because these oils are obtained by solvent extraction and then destroyed. This process destroys the benefic properties of the oil and thus they become ineffective. Using cold-pressed oil will ensure that the vitamins and therapeutic benefits of the oil are retained during manufacture.

The most common types of carrier oils are sweet almond, apricot kernel, grapeseed, avocado (both refined and unrefined), black seed, borage, calendula, coconut, jojoba, peach kernel, rose hip, St. John's wort, sunflower, peanut, olive, pecan, macadamia nut, sesame, evening primrose, walnut and wheat germ. Depending on the benefit that you are looking out for, choose your oil. These oils by themselves too have therapeutic properties. The carrier oils sold in the grocery store are not cold-pressed but are heated and hence have minimal therapeutic value. These oils should not be used in aromatherapy. Mineral oil should never be used in aromatherapy since it is not a natural product. It prevents the absorption of aromatherapy bath oil into the skin.

Unlike aromatherapy bath oils, carrier oils can go rancid. Always buy the natural and unadulterated oil. But you can buy oils with vitamin E added to it since vitamin E is the most popular natural preservative. The carrier oils should be light and non-sticky which makes their penetration into the skin very easy. Always purchase these oils from a reputed manufacturer. Take references of the experts in aromatherapy for good-quality brands before purchasing any carrier oil.

Almond oil (Sweet) - extracted from the kernel. Contains glycosides, minerals, vitamins and proteins. It is good for skin, helps to relieve itchiness, soreness, dryness and inflammation.

Apricot kernel oil - extracted from the kernel. Contains minerals, vitamins. Used for sensitive, dry, inflamed and all skin types, particularly for pre-matured age.

Avocado pear oil - extracted from the fruit. Contains vitamins, proteins, lecithin and fatty acids. Used in all skin types, especially dehydrated dry skin and eczema.

Carrot oil - contains vitamins, minerals and beta-carotene. Used when there is premature ageing, itching, eczema, dryness and psoriasis. Reduces scars and is very rejuvenating.

Corn oil - contains minerals, vitamins and protein. It is soothing for all types of skin.

Evening Primrose - contains vitamins, minerals and gamma linolenic acid. Used in menopause related tensions, multiple sclerosis, heart diseases. Used in the treatment of eczema and psoriasis. Prevents premature ageing of the skin.

Hazelnut oil - extracted from the kernel, contains vitamins, minerals and proteins. It has a slight astringent action and can be used for all skins.

Peanut oil, Safflower oil, Soya bean oil and Sunflower oil all contain vitamins, minerals and can be used for all types of skin.

Sesame oil - contains vitamins, minerals, protein, lecithin and amino acids and is useful in rheumatism, arthritis, eczema and psoriasis.

Essential Oil Inhalers

"Inhalers" the word brings to ones mind a running or a jammed nose, suffering from cold. To many the word is synonym to any branded product like Vicks inhaler. But actually inhalers are a portable device that gets the medicine directly in to the patient's lungs through breathing. One would be surprised to know that, to many they also serve one of the ways to take aromatherapy.

Aromatherapy heals people using the aroma of natural plants and herbs. Aromatherapy makes use of oils extracted from natural herbs and plants. These oils are known as aromatherapy oil or essential oil. There are many ways of taking aromatherapy like massage, inhaling the aroma, in bath water, dispensers, candles etc.. Inhaling aromatherapy oil affects the central nervous system through the olfactory system. Special inhalers are available in the market for inhaling the essential oil.

Aromatherapy using inhaler is mainly practiced for treating asthma. Essential oil inhalers are portable and could be carried in a pocket or could be hanged around the neck using a string. Using essential inhaler is very simple. Put 8 to 10 drops of desired essential oil or essential blend on a cotton ball and place the cotton ball in to the inhaler. Gently put the essential oil inhaler in one nostril while closing the other and inhale the aroma. Repeat the same procedure for the other nostril too.

Essential oil inhalers are reusable and seal tight and powerful. When the essential oil inhaler is not in use it must be kept inside its container tightly screwed, this will prevent the aroma from leaking out. Using inhalers avoids one from practicing the conventional way of inhaling, where in the patient use to add few drops of essential oil or essential blend to hot water and cover his face with a towel or blanket to inhale the hot vapours. Some of the essential oils or essential blends that could be used with essential oil inhalers are eucalyptus, lavender, chamomile, Rosemary etc. Eucalyptus could be used for treating cough and cold. Lavender could be used for treating insomnia.

As aromatherapy and the essential oils used are completely natural and herbal it does not have any negative side effects.

Hydrosols

The water left behind when you produce essential oil by the means of steam or water distillation is known as hydrosol. It is also called as floral water or distillate water. Since the water soluble parts of the plant are dissolved in this water, hydrosol too retains some of the therapeutic properties of the plant and can be used for healing purpose. Though this water is known as floral water or distillate water, this water can be produced from other parts of plant like herbs, pines, leaves, barks, woods and seeds.

Hydrosol has wonderful aroma of the parent plant. It contains the same therapeutic benefits of the plant. Some plants are specifically distilled for their hydrosol instead of making hydrosol a by-product of the extraction process of the plant. Always ask the seller the details about the hydrosol and try to get some samples before use. This is a crucial since today many hydrosols have synthetic compounds in them. This has caused skin irritation in the sensitive people. Also these compounds do not have any therapeutic properties. Some vendors may also sell water blended with essential oils as floral waters or hydrosols.

Original hydrosols have a wide range of therapeutic values since many active, water-soluble compounds of the plants are present in this water but not in the corresponding essential oil. Hence these floral waters can be used in a wide variety of ways like adding to the bath, sprayed across the room to freshen up your surroundings, to refresh and relax or in skincare products. You can make facial toners and other skin care products. Add them to bath for a refreshing experience or use as a light cologne or body spray. You can add a drop or two in a finger bowl for an elegant, romantic dinner. The common hydrosols are: rose, roman chamomile, chamomile german, peppermint, Melissa, orange blossom (neroli) and lavender.

These hydrosols can be used on the elderly and children or on people with sensitive skin. They can be used undiluted unlike essential oils. However, you should not take them internally. Always keep them away from the eyes.

Cooking and Baking with Pure Essential Oils

Since they are the plant products, essential oils contain practically all the minerals, vitamins and healing properties. They have the healing nutrients, oxygenating molecules, amino acid precursors, coenzyme A factors, trace minerals, enzymes, vitamins, hormones etc. that the parent plant contains. Also, being highly concentrated, they are more potent and have higher therapeutic powers that the plants or herbs from which they are derived. These oils do not lose their healing properties and oxygen molecules. The oils which are 100% pure essential oils and safe can be used for your daily cooking and home use. These oils are considered as food items and not as medicines by the government. The chemical structure of these oils is similar to that of our human tissues. This makes them compatible with human protein and the body identifies and absorbs them easily. This makes it easy for you to replace the hydrogenated vegetable oil used in baking of cookies, biscuits etc. with these essential oils.

The following are the tips to cook and bake with pure essential oils safely, while maintaining their healing properties:

- o To make a stronger spice oils like basil, cinnamon, marjoram, nutmeg, oregano, or thyme, dip a toothpick in the essential oil and stir it in the recipe after cooking.
- o Add 1 or 2 drops of lightly fragrant oil like citrus oils lemon, orange, tangerine before serving to prevent the oil from evaporating to make the recipe for 6-10 people.
- o Most of the oils are highly volatile and hence have to be added before serving. Some strong oils like basil, oregano and rosemary when simmered will produce a strong odour.
- o Dilute the essential oils with vegetable oil, agave syrup, almond or rice milk before use. Add 1 drop of essential oil to 1 teaspoon of hone, agave syrup or to 2 ounces of beverage.
- o Always use the therapeutic quality essential oils.

- o Use the cookware you are comfortable with.
- o Inhale the aroma of the oil 6 times a day to suppress appetite. It should be inhaled for a longer time. Brief inhaling will have the opposite effect of reversing the appetite. Change the oils daily for the best results.
- o Do not use microwave oven as it destroys the enzymes in the food and changes the frequency of the food.
- o Avoid using sugar, aspartame and other artificial sweeteners.
- o Make ginger cookies with ginger, cinnamon, clove and nutmeg.
- o Add lemon, orange, or tangerine oil to the sponge or bundt cake.
- o Add peppermint or spearmint oil to chocolate cake, brownie or frosting recipes.
- o Improve the taste of the pumpkin pie or spice cake by adding nutmeg, cinnamon, clove or ginger.
- o Make tomato sauces, pizza, ravioli, and lasagna recipes more healthy by adding oregano, marjoram, thyme, or basil.

Some common essential oil recipes for cooking:

- o *Salad Dressings or Salad Oils*—Lemon, lavender, rosemary, clove or peppermint in Vegetable Mixing Oil or Massage Oil Base.
- o *Meat and Sauces*—Basil, marjoram, oregano, or thyme.
- o *Cakes, Frosting, Puddings, Druit Pies*—Lemon, clove, orange, tangerine, or peppermint.
- o *Pie Crusts*—Vegetable Mixing Oil produces very flaky crusts.
- o *Herbal Teas*—Lavender, Roman chamomile, orange, tangerine, lemon, peppermint and melissa.
- o *Cool Refreshing Drinks*—Lemon, orange, tangerine, or peppermint added to a pitcher of cold water.
- o *Flavored Honey*—Cinnamon, clove, lavender, basil, chamomile or lemon. (Warm honey until it becomes a thin liquid then add the oil.)

Aromatheraphy

The word aromatherapy means "treatment using scents'. It refers to the use of essential oils in Holistic Healing to improve health and emotional well being and in restoring balance to the body. Essential oils are aromatic essences extracted from plants, flowers, trees, fruit, bark, grasses and seeds.

There are more than 150 types of oils that can be extracted. These oils have distinctive therapeutic, psychological and physiological properties that improve health and prevent illness. All essential oils have unique healing and valuable antiseptic properties. Some oils are anti-viral, anti-inflammatory, pain-relieving, anti-depressant, stimulating, relaxing, expectorating, support digestion and have diuretic properties too.

Essential oils get absorbed into our body and exert an influence on it. The residue gets dispersed from the body naturally. They can also affect our mind and emotions. They enter the body in three ways: by inhalation, absorption and consumption.

From the chemist's point of view, essential oils are a mixture of organic compounds viz., ketones, terpenes, esters, alcohol, aldehyde and hundreds of other molecules which are extremely difficult to classify, as they are small and complex. The essential oils' molecules are small. They penetrate human skin easily and enter the blood stream directly and finally get flushed out through our elementary system.

A concentrate of essential oils is not greasy; it is more like water in texture and evaporates quickly. Some of them are light liquid insoluble in water and evaporate instantly when exposed to air. It would take 100 kg of lavender to yield 3 kg of lavender oil; one would need 8 million jasmine flowers to yield barely I kg of jasmine oil.

Some of these aroma oils are very expensive. They are extracted using maceration. The purification process called defleurage is employed, and in some cases fat is used instead of oil. Then this process, called enfleurage, is used for final purification.

Some of the common essential oils used in aromatherapy for their versatile application are:

1. Clary Sage (Salvia Scarea)
2. Eucalyptus (Eucalyptus Globulus)
3. Geranium (Pelargonium Graveolens)
4. Lavender (Lavendula Vera Officinals)
5. Lemon (Citrus Limonem)
6. Peppermint (Mentha Piperita)
7. Petitgrain (Citus Aurantium Leaves)
8. Rosemary (Rosmarinus Officinals)
9. Tea-tree (Melaleuca Alternifolia)
10. Ylang Ylang (Cananga Odorata)

The oils mentioned can be good in a beginner's kit.

Origin of Aromatherapy

The oldest use of aroma oils is known to be as old as 6000 years back when Egyptian physician, Imhotep, the then God of Medicine and Healing recommended fragrant oils for bathing and massaging. In 4,500 B.C. Egyptians used myrrh and cedar wood oils for embalming their dead and 6,500 years later the preserved mummies prove the fact discovered by the modern researchers that the cedar wood contains natural fixative and strong anti-bacterial and antiseptic properties.

Hippocrates, the Greek father of Medicine, recommended regular aromatherapy baths and scented massages. This is what he effectively used to ward off plague from Athens. Romans utilised essential oils for pleasure and to cure pain and also for their popular perfumed baths and massages. Emperor New being indulgent in orgies, feasts and fragrances employed rose frequently to cure his headaches, indigestion and to maintain his high spirits while enjoying amusements.

During the great plague in London in 1665, people burnt bundles of lavender, cedar wood and cypress in the streets and carried posies of the same plants as their only defence to combat infectious diseases. Aromatherapy received a wider acceptance in the early twentieth century. In 1930s Rene-

Maurice-Gatte Fosse, a French chemist, diped his burnt hand in lavender oil. To his surprise the wound healed very quickly without any infection or scarring. He did considerable research on various oils and their therapeutic and psychotherapeutic properties.

Dr. Jean Volnet, French army surgeon extensively used essential oils in World War IL It was Madame Morquerite Murry who gave the holistic approach to aroma oils by experimenting with them for individual problems.

Today, research have proved the multiple use of aroma oils. Medical research in the recent years has uncovered the fact that the odours we smell have a significant impact on the way we feel. Smells act directly on the brain like a drug according to scientific research. For instance smelling lavender increases alpha wave frequency in the back of the head and this state is associated with relaxation.

Essential oils like spiritual healing (Reiki, Pranic, Magnified), homeopathic, herbal and flower remedies have a life force that vibrates within the body and the benefit exerted is too subtle to evaluate.

How does Aroma Oils Work?

Dr. Alan Huch, a neurologist, psychiatrist and also the director of Smell and Taste Research Centre in Chicago says, "'Smell acts directly on the brain, like a drug". Our nose has the capacity to distinguish 1,00,000 different smells, (many of which) affect us without our knowing about the same.

The aroma enters our nose and connects with cilia, the fine hair inside the nose lining. The receptors in the cilia are linked to the olfactory bulb which is at the end of the smell tract. The end of the tract is in turn connected to the brain itself. Smells are converted by cilia into electrical impulses that are transmitted to the brain through olfactory system.

All the impulses reach the limbic system. Limbic system is that part of the brain which is associated with our moods, emotions, memory and learning. All the smell that reaches the limbic system has a direct chemical effect on our moods.

For example smelling lavender increases alpha waves in the brain and it is this wave that helps us to relax. A whiff of jasmine increases beta waves in the brain and this wave is associated with an increased agile and alert state.

Limbic system is also a storehouse of millions of remembered smells. That is why the mere fragrance of haystack takes us back to childhood.

The molecular sizes of the essential oils are very tiny and they can easily penetrate through the skin and get into the blood stream. It takes anything between a few seconds to two hours for the essential oils to enter the skin and within 4 hours the toxins get out of the body through urine, perspiration and excreta.

Aroma oils work like magic for stress-related problems, psychosomatic disorders, skin infections, hair loss, inflammations, pains arising from muscular or skeletal disorders to name some of the application. Actually essential oils have innumerable applications.

In Bristol, lavender oil was used on 28 patients who had undergone by-pass surgery. 24 of them reported reduced breathing rates, lower blood pressure and anxiety levels.

In Paris, in 1985, 28 women were given treatment for thrush using essential oils. After 90 days the clinical examination showed that 21 of them had been cured completely.

Essential oils are safe to use. The only caution being they should never be used directly because some oils may irritate sensitive skin or cause photo-sensitivity. They should be blended in adequate proportion with the carrier oils. A patch test is necessary to rule out any reactions.

How to Use Aroma Oils?

Essential oils can be used in a variety of ways at home and place of work. Some of the common ways are:

Inhalation: Add 2-3 drops of essential oil depending on which oil you have selected to the hot boiling water and inhale the steam by covering your head with a towel to stop the steam from escaping. Steaming also helps open the pores of the skin and thus more oil is absorbed giving the additional benefit of a facial. The bowl which has the hot water and the aroma oil could be left under the bed so that the room is enveloped in aromatic fragrance. This could be done with the same bowl of hot steaming water and essential oil which had been used earlier for inhalation. A drop or two sprinkled on a handkerchief can give a lasting benefit of the aroma oil. For a very peaceful and relaxed sleep one or two drops of essential oils on a tissue kept inside the pillow or cushion could be used.

Diffusers and Vapourisers: Diffusers are generally made of ceramic or clay. The diffuser has a cave like opening to house small candles or earthen oil lamps and the top is shaped like a curved cup to hold a little water and few drops of aroma oil. Fill the top cup with water add a few drops of essential oils depending on the oil chosen then light the candle or the lamp.

For the oil lamp to last for a long duration, add castor oil to the earthen lamp because castor oil burns for a very long time as compared to the other oils used to light a lamp. Once the water and oil heat up, evaporation takes place and the whole atmosphere is filled with the aromatic scent. The process of evaporation continues for nearly five to six hours.

This is ideal for presenting a conducive ambience during a gathering or even in bedrooms, hotels, living -rooms, etc., and anywhere where scented air is required. One can get instant relief from pain a relaxed and positive feeling prevails when the right oil is used. One needs to be careful in choosing the right essential oil.

Vaporisers are the insect repellents used normally in the form of mats or other types of vaporisers kept for repelling insects. One could reuse the used mats by adding 2-3 drops of essential oil of your own choice and keeping them lit (electrically). Slowly the smell will get released and the area would be filled with soothing aroma. Lemon or rosemary are beneficial for offices, lavender for bedroom, antiseptic tea-tree for disinfecting a sick room and citronella for repelling the insects.

Massage: The most common form of treatment is massage because the dual benefits of touch therapy and scent therapy are simultaneously enjoyed. Massage improves the circulation of the blood, tones the muscles, detoxify toxins, releases trapped energy from tense muscles. The fragrance triggers a sense of pleasure and well being.

The penetration of essential oil through the skin during massages is high. Generally carrier oils like sunflower, coconut, olive, sweet almond, sesame and vegetable oils are mixed with aroma oils. The aroma oils should not be used for massages directly without dilution. About 10 drops or 1 teaspoon of essential oil can be mixed to about 30 ml of carrier oil. This makes a very rejuvenating massage oil.

Baths: This is an easy way to relax using essential oils.

Foot Bath: You can immerse your feet in a bowl of luke warm water to which 2-3 drops of essential oil is added. This is a very refreshing experience after a hard days work and if you have sweaty and smelly feet then too this foot bath is very profitable.

Pot Pourri: Pot Pourri as the name suggests is a mixture of dried flowers, herbs, grass and seed pods. Few drops of essential oil added to the pot pourri and kept in a bowl would keep giving out aromatic fragrance for 4-6 weeks. Another more effective method would be to keep the pot pourri mixture after adding the essential oil in a closed container overnight so that the oil gets absorbed. The following morning the box can be kept open and the lingering aroma would fill the area.

Bed Time: Sprinkle 2-3 drops on the pillow cover or on a tissue that can be placed under the pillow or cushion cover and inhaled just before sleeping or while sleeping. This can be very useful in treating headaches, stress, tension and in boosting confidence. Some of the essential oils act as an aphrodisiac too.

Compresses: Both cold and hot compresses are profitable. Add 2-3 drops of aroma oil to a bowl of hot (depending on how much of heat you can withstand) or warm water and dip a hand towel or piece of cotton to enable it to absorb the mixture then squeeze out the excess water and place the towel or cotton on the area to be treated. Leaving the compress on the area for 2 hours is quite beneficial. Oil like lavender is usually used. This provides relief when used over bruises, skin problems and pre menstrual syndromes.

To make cold compress, add 6 cubes of ice to a bowl with 2-3 drops of essential oil and dip a hand towel or a piece of cotton to absorb the mixture then squeeze out the excess water and place the towel or cotton on the area to be treated. Cold compress is highly helpful in treating burns, sore feet, hangover, sprains and headaches. After a facial the use of hot and cold compress alternately helps the skin.

Oral Intake: It is an accepted practice abroad to take essential oil orally as it is safe. However, care should be taken to take it only under the supervision or guidance of an experienced aromatherapy practitioner. Few oils can be taken internally in prescribed dosage for a particular problem like indigestion under the guidance of a qualified therapist only.

Beauty Treatment: Aroma oils have been used as an application for the skin from times immemorial. As they are highly soothing in treating and enhancing the natural beauty of the skin they can be safely incorporated in facials, massages, manicures, pedicures, scalp treatment, hair wash, hair treatment along with other creams and oils. Rose, chamomile, lemon, lavender, geranium, sandalwood are some good oils for facials irrespective of the fact that beauty treatment is given to normal, mature, dry, oily, sensitive or problem skin. Either one of these or a combination of two of them could be used. The carrier oils that are helpful in a beauty treatment are sweet almond, wheat germ, peach kernel, apricot kernel and sunflower. Steam facials with essential oils are also rejuvenating and help in improving the skin texture.

Room Sprays: There is a call for protecting the environment and this is becoming a prime concern worldwide. Aerosols are being discouraged due to their ozone depleting properties. Essential oils are natural and hence they could be used liberally to deodorise a room, freshen and scent your bathroom, living-room, bedroom, dining-room, office cabin, etc. Merely add 10-12 drops of aroma oil to half a litre of water and spray the mixture with the help of a spray bottle. Oils like lavender, lemon, peppermint, pine and rosemary are best for this application. Cupboards, wardrobes can also be disinfected. If a room smells of dampness or there are moulds in the hotel rooms, houses, offices or factories and shops the essential oil along with water can be sprayed.

Essential Oils and Culinary Herbs

Essential oil plants and culinary herbs include a broad range of plant species that are used for their aromatic value as flavourings in foods and beverages and as fragrances in pharmaceutical and industrial products. Essential oil plants derive from aromatic plants of many genera distributed worldwide. In the United States, the most economically important sources of domestically produced essential oils are industrial by-products from citrus, balsam fir, pine, and cedarwood, while the most important crops grown in the U.S. for essential oils are peppermint and spearmint. Most other essential oils used in the U.S. are imported at an annual cost in 1988 of $150 million (USDA 1989b).

Culinary herbs are herbaceous aromatic plants grown and marketed fresh or dried and include many of the same aromatic plants which are grown for their extractable essential oils. Significant quantities of dried culinary herbs are imported annually into the U.S. Recent estimates by the USDA Foreign Agricultural Service reported that more than $349 million of dried condiments, seasonings, and flavourings and $20 million of spice oleoresins were imported into the U.S. in 1988 (USDA 1989a). A significant amount of selected herbs are domestically produced for the dried spice or condiment market Domestic production of these and other herbs and spices now imported is increasing for both processing and fresh market.

The objectives of this paper are to provide an overview to the plants which are processed in the U.S. for essential oils and to identify fresh culinary herbs that are or can be grown in the continental U.S. The potential opportunities and constraints for production of these new crops in American agriculture will be highlighted.

Essential Oils

Chemistry and Extraction of Essential Oils

Essential oils are natural plant products which accumulate in specialized structures such as oil cells, glandular trichomes, and oil or resin ducts. The formation and accumulation of essential oils in plants have been reviewed by Croteau (1986), Guenther (1972) and Runeckles and Mabry (1973). Chemically, the essential oils are primarily composed of mono- and sesquiterpenes and aromatic polypropanoids synthesized via the mevalonic acid pathway for terpenes and the shikimic acid pathway for aromatic polypropanoids.

The essential oils from aromatic plants are for the most part volatile and thus, lend themselves to several methods of extraction such as hydrodistillation, water and steam distillation, direct steam distillation, and solvent extraction (ASTA 1968, Guenther 1972, Heath 1981, Sievers 1928). The specific extraction method employed is dependent upon the plant material to be distilled and the desired end-product. The essential oils which impart the distinctive aromas are complex mixtures of organic constituents, some of which being less stable, may undergo chemical alterations when subjected to high temperatures.

In this case, organic solvent extraction is required to ensure no decomposition or changes have occurred which would alter the aroma and fragrance of the end-product. Newer methods of essential oil extraction such as using supercritical CO2 which yield very high quality oils are commercially used, but are less common and beyond the financial means of most processors.

The recovery of nonvolatile essential oils are also obtained by solvent extraction although the process is more difficult and complex than the recovery of the volatiles. This process yields an aromatic resinous product known as an oleoresin, which is more concentrated than an essential oil and which has wide application in the food industry (Heath 1981).

Essential Oils as Industrial By-products

Although a primary focus of this review is to highlight aromatic plants and culinary herbs produced in the U.S., it is important to recognize that the largest quantities of essential oils produced in the U.S. are actually by-products from industrial processes yielding higher value primary products. Citrus essential oils are recovered from the peel which contain the oil sacs or glands located irregularly in the outer mesocarp of the fruit (Matthews and Braddock 1987). These glands are embedded at different depths in the flavedo, the coloured, outer portion of the fruit and must be removed by first rupturing the glands by pressure or mechanical rasping (Matthews and Braddock 1987).

The recovery of citrus oils by mechanical expression is generally obtained by two types of commercial extractors, the FMC Citrus juice Extractor (FMC Corp.) and the Brown Extractor (Automatic Machinery Corp.) (Kealey and Kinsella 1979, Kesterson et al. 1971). Citrus oils are recovered as cold-pressed oils or as a specific constituent such a d-limonene as by-products of the juice and beverage industry and yield important aromatic and flavoring compounds used in a wide array of food, cosmetic and industrial products.

The other large quantity of essential oils produced as industrial by-products in this country comes from the wood and pulp manufacturing industries. More than 1650 tonnes of such oils, predominantly from cedarwood, are produced annually (Lawrence 1979).

Essential Oil Plants

In the United States, only a relatively few plant species are now cultivated and produced for essential oils. The most important species includes the mints. The production and processing of mint in the United States has a rich history (Landing 1969, Rabak 1916) and is the most mechanized system of essential oil production in the world (Ellis 1937, Ellis et al. 1941; Green 1975, 1963, Lacy 1981, Smith and Robertson 1941). Mint oils are obtained by steam distillation.

The only other essential oil crop in the United States of significant volume is dill where the oils are used in the manufacture of pickles. Although dill oil can be obtained from the steam distillation of either seeds or foliage, it is often obtained by harvesting dill as a green herb after the seeds have formed but have not yet ripened. Dill seed oil is from the seeds and dill weed oil is from the green herb prior to flowering (Heath 1981).

While many other herbs have been produced for essential oil in limited quantities, a complete list of crop species and production area is difficult to obtain and confirm. Most all the essential oils derived from temperate zone aromatic plants currently imported could be produced for essential oil domestically. However, opportunities for domestic production are limited because most essential oils from traditional herbs have limited markets making penetration into established markets very difficult.

Many buyers and users have little interest in changing their suppliers unless supplies from abroad become limited due to political instability, contamination (such as the Chernobyl release of radioactive materials), or crop failure which permits new suppliers into the marketplace. An additional difficulty in establishing new sources of traditional essential oils is in demonstrating the ability to produce the quantity and quality demanded by the industry at a competitive price.

Many countries have government funded programmes to establish new industries for export and which absorb much of the developmental costs associated with the evaluation and introduction of new crops. When these programmes are coupled with crop champions and a strong relationship with the processing industry, the success of new crop development significantly increases. Such a programme encouraged extensive work with several herbs for potential production in the prairies of western Canada (Embong et al. 1977a-e). Such programmes have allowed Israel to go from an importer to a significant exporter of essential oils (128 tonnes of essential oils annually) in a relatively short time period (Putievsky 1989).

International development programmes have also contributed to the creation of essential oil industries. Technical assistance and funding from the Marshall Plan, enabled the large scale cultivation of herbs, spices and medicinal plants in Hungary (Mathe 1989). Prior to WWII, most Hungarian herbs were collected from the wild, but in part as a result of such an economic development programme, Hungary has emerged as a significant exporter of cultivated essential oils (65,808 tonnes produced in 1982).

One of the challenges in developing new essential oil crops or in establishing a new geographical area for the production of an essential oil already on the market is procuring or developing generic lines with the suitable agronomic characteristics and desirable chemical constituents. The evaluation of a large and diverse germplasm collection thus becomes the first step in new crop development. This stage alone could take many years unless a processor supplies the particular chemotype that meets their processing needs. Unlike peppermint which must be vegetatively propagated, most essential oil crops are open pollinated and available seed have not been selected for homogeneity in growth or for flavor and aroma. Two examples will suffice to illustrate both the chemical diversity of herb cultivars and germplasm and approaches to crop improvement.

Parsley oil: Little information was available on the compounds responsible for the flavor of parsley and the genetic variability of the essential oil constituents of this important culinary herb. A recent study showed that essential oil content of a large germplasm collection ranged from 0.00 to 0.16% (v/ fresh weight) and that the oil constituents varied significantly although the major constituent was 1,3,8-p-menthatriene, followed by ß-phellandrene, myristicin, and myrcene (Simon and Quinn 1988). In parallel study evaluating the essential oils of commercially available parsley curly-leaf types had as high essential oil content as the flat-leaf types, commonly believed to be more flavourful (Simon et al. 1989).

Basil Oil: Sweet basil (Ocimum basilicum L.) is a popular culinary herb and a source of essential oils (ITC 1986) extracted by steam distillation from the leaves and flowering tops and used to flavor foods, in dental and oral products, and in fragrances. There are several types of basil oil on the world market European, French, or sweet basil; Egyptian; Reunion or Comoro; Bulgarian; and Java (Heath 1981). The European basil oils, considered to be the highest quality, contain methyl chavicol d-linalool and to a lesser extent 1,8-cineole, plus many other compounds (Guenther 1985, Simon et al. 1984). Egyptian basil oil is similar to the European, except that the concentration of d-linalool is lower and methyl chavicol is higher. Reunion or Comoro contains little d-linalool, but has a very high concentration of methyl chavicol (Lawrence et al. 1972, Simon et al. 1984). Bulgarian basil oil is rich in methyl-cinnamate and Java basil oil is rich in eugenol (Heath 1981).

From an evaluation of the entire USDA collection plus other commercial and wild sources, we observed a wide range of chemical variation within O. basilicum and other species (O. canum, O. sanctum, O. gratissimum, and O. kilimand-scharicum). We have identified chemotypes that represent each of the commercial types of basil oil. Promising lines are being screened for chemical stability, vigor, and uniformity. The characteristics of the population has continued to improve under mass selection. Isolation blocks serve as seed sources. We are currently developing a new line rich in methyl cinnamate (Simon et al. 1990).

Prospects

Market surveys have reviewed world production of essential oils and identified areas of future growth (Greenhalgh 1979, Lawrence 1985, ITC 1986). For essential oil crops to be successfully developed in the United States, a long term coordinated strategy is required with either strong support from industry and grower groups or significant support by state and/or federal programmes in concert with growers and the users of essential oils.

Regions where the industrial infrastructure already exists (*e.g.* extraction equipment growers familiar with essential oil production, with brokers, buyers and processors in the proximity) will have the greatest opportunities and chance of success in developing new essential oil crops into American agriculture. New essential oil crops must be compatible with existing crops in a farm operation and offer economic returns at levels higher than those presently received.

Successful introduction of new plant sources of raw aroma chemicals for the fragrance industry could allow the rapid development of a new industry. An example is the development through selection of Monarda spp. rich in geraniol in Morden, Manitoba (Rafe Guadiel, personal communication) or Ocimum spp. rich in methyl cinnamate or methyl chavicol (Simon et al. 1990). The creation of new markets for specialized oils can take many years and would be most successful when working in collaboration with an end-user whose needs can be met by the new product.

The incorporation of new aromas into perfumes and fragrances and the development of new products is critical to the success of the perfumer and flavor chemist. The difficulty for the agricultural researcher is to learn the types of aromas and chemical constituents desired by the perfumer and flavorist. The identification of new species rich in desirable essential oils may be a promising route to pursue.

Bibliography

Adams H.: *Hot Pepper Improvement*, St. Michael, CARDI, 1997.

Agarwal P. K.: *Improvement of Citrus*, New Delhi, Malhotra Publishing House, 1993.

Alexander M. P. and Ganeshan S.: *Pollen Storage*, New Delhi, Malhotra Publishing House, 1993.

Andrews J.: *The Domesticated Capsicums*, University of Texas Press. 1995.

Andrews L.: *Citrus Production - Orange*, St. Augustine, Trinidad and Tobago, 1990

————: *Production of Minor Crops Sapodilla, Tamarind, Guava and Genip*, Port of Spain, Trinidad and Tobago, 1996.

Arguello D. S.: *Production, Post-harvest Management and Exportation of Tropical Fruits in Costa Rica*, Wageningen, Technical Centre for Agricultural and Rural Cooperation, 1992.

Ashworth S.: *Seed to Seed*, Decorah, Seed Savers Publications, 1991.

Barbeau G.: *Tropical Fruits in Nicaragua*, Managua, Nicaragua Ministerio de Desarrollo Agropecuario, Agraria, 1990.

Batlle I. and Tous J.: *Carob Tree (Ceratonia siliqua L.)*. Rome, International Plant Genetic Resources Institute, 1997.

Berger, P.L.: *Pyramids of Sacrifice: Political Ethics and Social Change*, New York, Basic Books, 1974.

————: *Pyramids of Sacrifice: Political Ethics and Social Change*, New York, Basic Books, 1974.

Brooks, D.: *Water: Local-Level Management*, Ottawa, International Development Research Centre, 2002.

Bunnik J. S. C.: *Fresh Fruits and Vegetable: a Survey on the Netherlands and other Major Markets in the European*

Community, Netherlands, Centre for the Promotion of Imports from Developing Countries, 1990.

Burton W.G.: *The Potato*, Holland, H. Veenman & Zonen N.V., 1966.

Cao Van P.: *An Integrated Approach for the Production and Processing of Minor Fruits in Martinique (FWI)*, Port of Spain, Trinidad and Tobago, 1996.

Cardona M. J. G., Carvajal S. L. B., Salinas D. G. C. and Isaza R. G. B. : *Proceedings of the International Seminar on Plantain Production, Quindio, Colombia,* Quindio, Corporation Colombiana de Investigation Agropecuaria, 1998.

Chadha K. L. and Pareek O. P.: *Advances in Horticulture: Fruit Crops,* New Delhi, Malhotra Publishing House, 1993.

Chambers, R.: *Rural Development: Putting the Last First*, London, Longman, 1983.

Collymore L.: *Fruit Production in Barbados*, Port of Spain, Trinidad and Tobago, 1996.

Coste R.: *Coffee: the Plant and the Product*, London, MacMillan, 1992.

Crucefix D.: *Avocado Variety Selection for Export Development,* Roseau, CARDI, 1996.

Cull Brian & Lindsay Pax: *Fruit Growing in Warm Climates for Commercial Growers & Home Gardeners*, Australia, Reed Books, 1995.

Currah L. and Proctor F. J.: *Onions in Tropical Regions*, Kent, Natural Resources Institute, 1990.

Daniells J.: *Illustrated Guide to the Identification of Banana varieties in the South Pacific*, Canberra, ACIAR, 1995.

Degras L.: *Yam: a Tropical Root Crop*, Wageningen, CTA/ MacMillan, 1993.

Dhatt A. S. and Singh Z.: *Propagation and Rootstocks of Citrus*, New Delhi, Malhotra Publishers, 1993.

Diederichsen A.: *Coriander (Coriandrum sativum L.).* Rome, International Plant Genetic Resources Institute, 1996.

Doijode S. D.: *Seed Germination in Fruits*, New Delhi, Malhotra Publishers, 1993.

Dudley, E.: *The Critical Villager: Beyond Community Participation*, London, Routledge, 1993.

Featherly H. I.: *Taxonomic Terminology of the Higher Plants*, USA, Iowa State College Press, 1954.

Ferentinos L.: *Proceeding of the Sustainable Taro Culture for the Pacific Conference*, Honolulu, HITAHR, 1993.

Forde S: *Proceedings of CARDI / CTA Workshop on Marketability of Caribbean Minor Fruits*, Port of Spain, Trinidad and Tobago, 1996.

Georges, S.: *The Debt Boomerang: How Third World Debt Harms Us All*, Boulder, Westview Press, 1992.

Glowinski Louis: *The Complete Book of Fruit Growing in Australia*, Australia, Lothian Publishing Company Pty. Ltd., 1991.

Godden G.: *Growing Citrus Trees*, Australia, Lothian Publishing Company Pvt. Ltd., 1988.

Gowen S.: *Banana and Plantains*, London, Chapman Hall, 1996.

Green S.K. and Kim J. S.: *Sources of Resistance to Viruses of Pepper (Capsicum spp.): a Catalogue*, Taipei, AVRDC, 1994.

Gunjate R. T. and Tawde A. B.: *Propagation and Rootstocks of Mango*, New Delhi, Malhotra, 1993.

Hartley W.: *A Checklist of Economic Plants in Australia*, Melbourne, C.S.I.R.O., 1979.

Harwood, R. R.: *Marshalling Technology for Development: Proceedings of a Symposium*, Washington, DC, National Academy Press, 1995.

Herklots G. A. C.: *Vegetables in South East Asia*, London, George Allen & Unwin Ltd., 1972.

Hessayon D. G. Dr.: *The Vegetable Expert*, England, PBI, Publications, 1985.

Huaman Z.: *Descriptors for Sweet Potato*, Rome, International Board for Plant Genetic Resources, 1991.

Hurst Jacqui & Rutherford Lyn.: *A Gourmet's Book of Mushrooms & Truffles*, Sydney, Golden Press Pvt. Ltd., 1991.

Jacquat Christiane: *Plants from the Markets of Thailand*, Bangkok, Duang Kamol, 1990.

Jeffers P.: *Evaluation of Four Onion Varieties in Montserrat*, Plymouth, CARDI, 1992.

Kenridge K. C. and Hardy B.: *Biology and Agronomy of Forage Arachis*, Cali, International Centre for Tropical Agriculture, 1994.

Kroll R.: *Cut Flowers*, Wageningen, CTA, 1995.

Kunelius T.: *Annual Ryegrasses in Atlantic Canada*, Ottawa, Agriculture Canada, 1991.

Lofgren, H., Richards, A.: *Food Security, Poverty, and Economic Policy in the Middle East and North Africa*, Washington, DC, International Food Policy Research Institute, 2003.

Mabberley D. J.: *The Plant-Book : a Portable Dictionary of the Vascular Plants*, Cambridge, Cambridge University Press, 1997.

Madulid Domingo A.: *A Pictorial Cyclopedia of Philippine Ornamental Plants*, Philippines, Makati Metro Manila, 1995.

Malins A.: *Postharvest Handling of Pineapple and Mango*, Port of Spain, Trinidad and Tobago, 1992.

Mannetje, L. T. & Jones, R. M.: *Plant Resources of South-East Asia,* Wageningen, Pudoc Scientific Publishers, 1992.

Matsuoka H.: *Cultivation of Panicum Genetic Resources for Evaluation of Characteristics*, Tokyo, JICA, 1997.

Mc Donald F.: *Plant Tissue Culture Manual for Yam, Cassava, Sweet Potato, Dasheen (taro) and Tannia (cocoyam)*, Roseau, Dominica and Cave Hill, 1993.

Mellor, J. W.: *The New Economics of Growth*, Ithaca, Cornell University Press, 1976.

Miller William: *Dictionary of English Plant Names*, London, John Murray, 1884.

Mitra S.: *Postharvest Physiology and Storage of Tropical and Subtropical Fruits*, Oxon, CABI, 1997.

Morris M. L. : *Maize Seed Industries in Developing Countries*, Colorado, Lynne Rienner, 1998.

Morton Julia F.: *Fruits of Warm Climates*, Miami, Julia F. Morton Publisher, 1987.

Murali T. P. and Duncan E. J.: *In Vitro Propagation of Banana through Aseptic Manipulation of Male Inflorescences*, Port of Spain, NIHERST, 1990.

Nabhan G. P.: *Wild Phaseolus Ecogeography in the Sierra Madre Occidental, Mexico: Areographic Techniques for Targeting and Conserving Species Diversity*, Rome, International Board for Plant Genetic Resources, 1990.

Nijdam J. & De Jong A.: *Elsevier's Dictionary of Horticulture in Nine Languages*, Elsevier Scientific Publishing Co. Amsterdam; New York.

Oka H. I.: *Origin of Cultivated Rice*, Elsevier, Japan Scientific Societies Press, 1988.

Oldham P.: *Cost of Production of Major Tree Crops in Dominica*, Roseau, Ministry of Agriculture, 1991.

Ou Yang Jue Ya: *Comparative Study of Mandarin and Cantonese*, Beijing, China Social Sciences Publishing House, 1993.

Percival John: *The Wheat Plant - A Monograph*, London, Duckworth & Co., 1921.

Pilgrim R.: *Post Harvest Handling of Minor Exotics*, St. George's, Grenada, 1996.

Ragone D.: *Breadfruit: Artocarpus Altilis (Parkinson) Fosberg*, Rome, International Plant Genetic Resources Institute, 1997.

Rehm Sigmund: *Multilingual Dictionary of Agronomic Plants*, Boston, Kluwer Academic Publishers, 1994.

Roy S. K.: *Research on Multipurpose Tree Species in Asia: In Vitro Clonal Propagation of Artocarpus Heterophyllus*, Bangkok, Winrock International Institute for Agricultural Development, 1991.

Singh H. P. and Chadha K. L.: *Genetic Resources of Citrus*, New Delhi, Malhotra Publishing House, 1993.

Sinha G. C., Reddy Y. T. N. and Singh G.: *Propagation and Rootstocks in Guava*, New Delhi, Malhotra Publishers, 1993.

Sperling L. and Berkowitz P. *Partners in selection: bean breeders and women bean experts in Rwanda*. Washington, USA: CGIAR, 1994.

Sreekumar V., Indrasenan G and Mammen G.: *Studies of the Quantitative and Qualitative Attributes of Ginger Cultivars*, Calicut, Kasaragod, 1990.

Stover R. H. and Simmonds N. W.: *Bananas*, United Kingdom: Longman Scientific and Technical, 1991.

Thavarasook C.: *Proceedings of the Mungbean Meeting 90, Chiang Mai, Thailand,* Bangkok, Tropical Agricultural Research Centre, 1991.

Thomas E.: *Fruit Production in St. Kitts and Nevis*, Port of Spain, IICA, 1996.

Vargas E. M., Macaya G., Baudoin J. P. and Rocha O. J.: *Variation in the Content of Phaseolin in Wild Populations of Lima Beans (Phaseolus lunatus L.) in the Central Valley of Costa Rica*. Plant Genetic Resources Newsletter, 2000.

Webb M.: *Weed Problems and their Control in Rice, Papaya, Citrus and Sugar cane: a Report to the Belize Plant Protection Service*, United Kingdom, Natural Resources Institute, 1993.

Whealy K.: *The Garden Seed Inventory*, Decorah, Seed Saver Publications, 1988.

Whitwell A.: *Dominica Orchard Crop Management and Research Project: Pest and Disease Management*, United Kingdom, Natural Resources Institute, 1991.

Woolfe Jennifer A.: *The Potato in the Human Diet*, Cambridge, Cambridge University Press, 1989.

Yoshida T.: *Cultivation of Citrus Genetic Resources for Evaluation of Characteristics*, Tokyo, JICA, 1996.

Index

A

B

C

D

E

F

R

S

T

U

V

W

Y

❑❑❑